NO MORE ILLNESS

Life after autoimmune disease

Written by Davida van der Walt

November 2019

Dedicated to every author cited in this book, who has gone to great lengths to educate people on how they can take responsibility for their health. And to every person with an autoimmune disease who has taken the bull by the horns and arrested their illness through lifestyle and diet changes. I salute you.

For information contact:
Davida van der Walt
Davida@on-route.co.za
www.on-route.co.za
+27 83 287 6015

DISCLAIMER - The information provided in this book, No More Illness, is for general information purposes and educational purposes only, aimed at improving lifestyle choices. All information is provided in good faith; however, we make no representation or warranty of any kind, express or implied, regarding accuracy, adequacy, validity, availability or completeness of any information. Under no circumstance shall we have any liability to you. The book does not contain any medical advice. Accordingly, before taking any actions based upon such information, we encourage you to consult with the appropriate medical professionals. The use or reliance of any information contained in this book is solely at your own risk.

FOREWORD

As a Homoeopath of over 25 years I have found Davida's book "No More Illness" an invaluable, well researched, holistic resource.

I treat many people with the symptoms Davida lists and I have found that lifestyle changes, renewing the gut and regular detoxing are the solutions to health and over all wellbeing. No longer can we take the advice of 'the powers that be' for our wellbeing, we must take responsibility for ourselves. This excellent book will support your lifestyle changes with this step by step, easy to follow system of renewing your health and therefore the health of the world.

As Davida says YOUR HEALTH IS YOUR GREATEST WEALTH.

Rebecca Sturgeon, LCPH

November 2019

THE REALITY OF MODERN LIFE

Are you constantly feeling tired and worn out? Battling with vague symptoms such as fatigue, bloating, aches and pains? Those are symptoms of modern life! We are so frustrated...we do not feel well, and when we visit our GP, we are given steroids, pain killers and acid blockers. Yet, we never really feel better.

What would it take for you to stop and think about why you are not feeling well? Do you not want to address the root cause? It is sad that we do not realise we are hurting ourselves.

After feeling lousy for years and not knowing what was wrong, I got very ill. At this point I was brought to an abrupt halt. I was diagnosed with Graves' Disease, which is an autoimmune disease that attacks the thyroid. I was advised to have radio-active iodine treatment. Little did I know what it would do to me. I got even worse. It is only then, when no medical doctors could help me, that I started doing my own research and a light bulb went on. What did I learn in this process?

Nothing we eat is real anymore

Have you taken the time to read food labels? Everything is processed. All the foods we love so much are loaded with preservatives to give a longer shelf life, or flavourants and colourants to make it taste better. Not to even mention MSG, fillers and binders. Reality is our bodies are not designed to cope with excess crap. Yes crap, that is what it is!

What about your veggies and fruits?

Most vegetables we buy are soaked in glyphosate, which is a pesticide. Glyphosate damages you stomach lining and causes havoc in your body! If that is not enough, most of our fruit and vegetables are genetically modified. Watch out for the term GMO on your food labels ~ it means genetically modified organisms. Wheat and oats are also genetically modified. This means that pesticides, such as glyphosate, are built into their DNA. Most seeds we buy today are GMO. Scary!

Meat or hormones?

Again, the meat we eat is injected with hormones and steroids to facilitate quick growth of the animals. By eating a lot of meat, you are absorbing these hormones. Does it now make sense why so many people battle with unexplained hormone imbalances?

Oh how I love my bread!

We eat excessive amounts of processed flours that contains gluten. Gluten generally refers to alpha gliadin gluten, which is gluten associated with wheat. Gluten is a family of proteins found in grains. All grains, by definition, have a different form of gluten. It is quite scary that the damage of the gut lining caused by gluten as well as other factors, can directly lead to malabsorption of nutrients. Most people, when they stop eating gluten-based products such as bread and wheat-based pasta, never need to use antacids again in their lives.

Stuck behind the computer

We have become dormant, indoor creatures. Lack of movement or exercise means that none of your organs work as they should. Oxygen does not flow freely through your body. This not only affects your body's ability to function, but also your body's ability to detox, and your brain's ability to function.

Furthermore, because we are stuck indoors, we do not see the sun anymore. Sun plays a key role in health, and, in particular, provides your body with Vitamin D that is fundamental to energy and good health.

Can't live without my cell phone

Electromagnetic frequencies (EMF) are everywhere. You can't go anywhere without exposure to harmful electromagnetic fields. Your cell phone radiates EMF, so does your WiFi, your microwave etc. This issue has gained much attention in the United States where people like Devra Davies are doing research on EMF and the effect on health, in particular as a cause of tumours.

Lack of sleep

For the body to recover effectively and the liver to excrete toxins effectively, we need enough sleep, and especially Rapid Eye Movement (REM) sleep. Due to many reasons, we do not sleep enough, or have low quality sleep. One reason is that we sleep with our phones right next to our beds. Cell phones and other electronic equipment, such as tablets and televisions, give off what is known as blue light. Blue light can inhibit the production of the sleep-inducing hormone melatonin and disrupt our sleeping patterns.

Environmental toxins hidden everywhere

The body is like a sponge, it absorbs everything through the biggest organ, namely the skin, as well as the lungs. Once again, we are oblivious to all the environmental toxins we are exposed to on a daily basis: from exhaust fumes, to personal care products, and a big culprit being household cleaning chemicals.

We do not know what we do not know

The biggest favour you can do for yourself, is to empower yourself with knowledge. What I learned on my journey is that there are many people out there that know the truth. And the truth is you need not feel "old" or ill. You can be well, and you can be vibrant!

The only thing between you and excellent health is your lack of knowledge. Sadly, this includes the medical fraternity. They get on average a few hours of nutrition training throughout their education.

I've learned that what you eat and what you expose yourself to can have a massive impact on your health. **I've learned that by addressing the root cause, you can be well!** Today I feel blessed that I claimed my life back. I want to help you do the same...

PREFACE

Introduction

The purpose of this book is to share the truth with you...the truth about health and wellness. The truth that what you put into your body and expose your body to can either make you ill or ensure great health.

My first book, No More Stress, was aimed at guiding you on how to proactively manage the impact of stress on your life.

This book is focused on how you can prevent illness through lifestyle changes. If you have been diagnosed with an autoimmune disease, this book will change your life forever. Even if you do not have an autoimmune disease, but just can't remember when last you felt well, this book will help you change your lifestyle so that you can claim your health and your life back. I want you to be empowered when it comes to your health. Know that your gut health is fundamental to your overall health. Heal your gut and your whole body heals.

I want you to feel so vibrant that you would want to jump out of bed in the morning and embrace your day.

For whom is the book intended?

This book is aimed at anyone who feels ill. You may just suffer from vague symptoms such as fatigue and muscle aches and pains. Or you could be diagnosed with an autoimmune disease. Do not let this opportunity pass to take charge of your health. Do not believe the lies that there is nothing you can do! There is plenty you can do...let me guide you through the process.

Commit to your journey and rediscover the energetic, healthy you! And guess what, an awesome advantage will be to get rid of brain fog and lose weight!

Layout of the book

Section 1   Introduction 10

Section 2   The root cause! 13

Section 3   Leaky gut or gut permeability 36

Section 4   Autoimmune disease, including diabetes 49

Section 5   Mood disorders 54

Section 6   Stubborn fat and heart disease 58

Section 7   Brain degeneration 67

Section 8   Skin disorders, allergies & MCS........................71

Section 9   Hormone imbalances 78

Section 10   Functional medicine 82

Section 11   Life style changes 86

Section 12   Remove the triggers 91

Section 13   Replace the bad with the good 116

Section 14   Reinculate the gut 137

Section 15   Repair the gut 142

Section 16   Rebalance your life 155

Section 17   Detox your environment 198

Section 18   Delicious and healthy recipes 218

Section 19   Food is medicine 227

Section 20   A glimpse of my journey 240

Section 21   In summary – what now? 255

ABOUT THE AUTHOR

Davida van der Walt

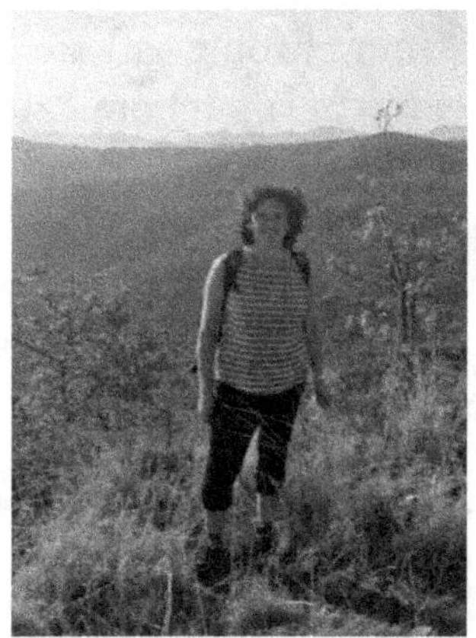

I am an industrial psychologist with a passion for wellness. Besides my experience addressing the softer issues on projects, I facilitate life strategy workshops and conduct life coaching where I share the principles captured in this book. My personal experience with an autoimmune disease and recovering from it to the extent that I am in remission, puts me in a unique position to share what works and what doesn't.

My aim is to empower you to take charge of your life, your thoughts, your decisions and your health. I read many health journals and sometimes must read an article five times to understand the content. My aim is to write this book in simple terms and language that everyone can understand. I sincerely hope that you find this book of interest and that it provides you with the tools to take responsibility for your health.

Davida van der Walt

December 2019

    Your Greatest Wealth is your Health

Section 1

Introduction

WHO IS THIS GUIDE FOR?

This guide is for everyone out there suffering from chronic fatigue, allergies, bloatedness, acid reflux and heart burn, chemical sensitivities, unexplained weight gain, as well as chronic aches and pains as a result of inflammation. If you are suffering from **ANY** chronic disease or autoimmune disease, then this guide is for you! It thus includes those of you suffering from fibromyalgia. We are so frustrated...we do not feel well, and when we visit our GP, we are given steroids, pain killers and acid blockers. Yet, we never really feel better. The medicine we take just causes secondary problems. If you are sick of feeling sick, then this is where you need to be. Dorland's Medical Dictionary defines health as "optimal physical, mental, and social well-being — not merely the absence of disease and infirmity." **I want you to be HEALTHY in the true sense of the word.**

Do note, I am not a doctor, I am a Life Style Coach focusing on HEALTH. The information provided in this programme is not medical advice. This programme is best followed working in conjunction with a Integrative Medicine or Functional Medicine practitioner that can treat infections or other medical illnesses. The programme is comprised of lifestyle changes that are tried and tested by myself and that I know work. My passion is to help others by sharing what I have learned on my own journey. It took me three years of research to get to this point.

I was diagnosed with Graves' Disease in 2015. Graves is an autoimmune disease which attacks the thyriod. I received radio-active iodine and was very sick for a long time. The first year I could not work full-time. I was barely able to work 2-3 hours a day.

The physician and specialist that administered the radio-active iodine left me to the wolves. Furthermore, my GP told me nothing was wrong with me. This whilst my whole body was inflamed. If you are not well and a doctor tells you that there is nothing wrong with you, do not

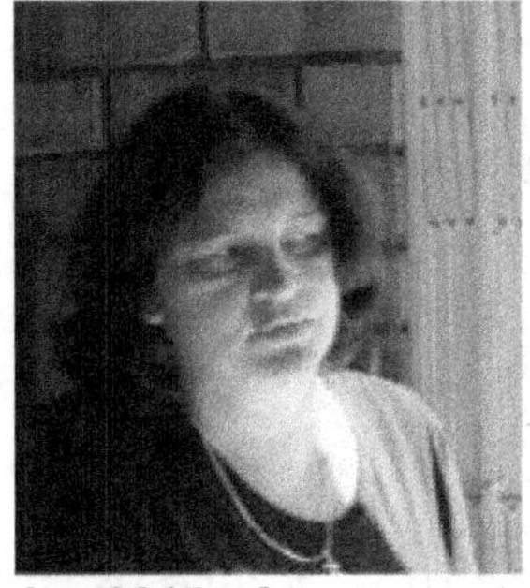

Jun 2015 - At my worst

ignore what your gut tells you! I then decided to take charge of my life and my health. I did extensive research and soon realised I needed to focus on healing my gut and building my immune system. In doing my research, I was astonished at how toxic our lives are. Not only do we think toxic thoughts, we also live in a toxic environment and lavish our bodies on a daily basis with even more toxins through what we eat, drink, and rub onto our skin. My journey taught me that **HEALTH STARTS IN THE GUT, BUT ALSO THAT NO SINGLE INTERVENTION IS ENOUGH**. A holistic approach is needed. Here you can see my improvement from June 2015 to November 2017.

In this programme, I will first help you understand why our lifestyle contributes to our illness. Thereafter we will follow the 5R's to get to a point of ultimate health!

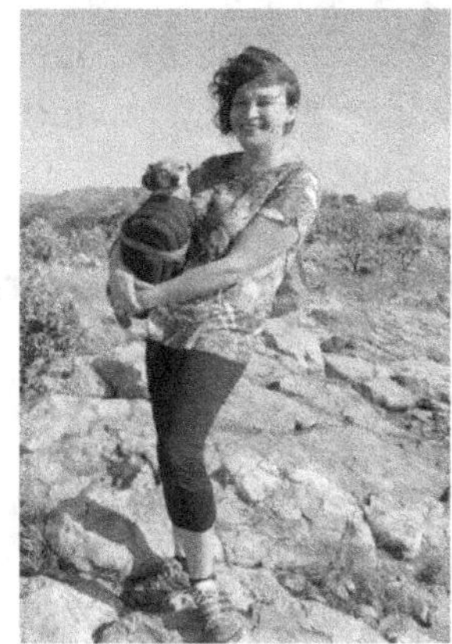

Nov 2017 - Healthy and energised!

R – Remove the triggers

R – Replace the bad with the good

R – Reinoculate your gut

R – Repair your gut

R – Rebalance your Life

I will guide you through a step-by-step process to use these 5Rs to regain your health.

 Your Greatest Wealth is your Health 11

Before we get into the nuts and bolts, note that this guide forms part of the CLAIM YOUR LIFE BACK PROGRAMME. Once you enroll to the Programme, you will have access to electronic meetings every second week, weekly educational e-mails that will guide you through a step-by-step process, as well as a WhatsApp group and Facebook group where you can enjoy the support of like-minded people. You can also pose personal questions via e-mail. These structures are put in place to provide you with the support and encouragement you would need throughout this journey. As this programme is dynamic, you will also receive regular updates via e-mail on any new additions to the programme.

If you only bought this book, you are losing out big time! I encourage you to reconsider and join the full programme. We all need a cheer leader. If you wish to enroll, please go to www.on-route.co.za.

Your decision to read this book and make the neccesray lifestyle changes is a commitment to your health and your future. This journey will be a lifelong journey. Every day you will explore new habits that will work for you, and some that won't. Embrace this journey. Do not resist change.

This book will transform your life forever!

Are you ready?

Section 2
The Root Cause

WHY ARE WE FEELING SICK?

Sick of being sick …

Dr Mark Hyman (https://drhyman.com/) says people often don't even know that their health condition is an autoimmune disease. He highlights that the list below all fall under the epidemic of autoimmunity:

- Cancer and post-cancer illnesses
- Depression
- Anxiety
- Multiple Sclerosis
- Celiac Disease
- Crohn's Disease
- Endometriosis
- Fibromyalgia
- Graves' Disease
- Hashimoto's Thyroiditis
- Lupus
- Chronic Fatigue
- Lyme Disease
- Peripheral Neuropathy
- Psoriasis
- Rheumatoid Arthritis
- Psoriatic Arthritis
- Raynaud's Phenomenon
- Restless Legs Syndrome (RLS)
- Scleroderma
- Ulcerative Colitis (UC)
- Brain disorders like Parkinson's and Alzheimer's

Others include a long list of symptoms like joint pain and even migraine headaches – so called "simple" conditions that ruin lives.

By following the guidelines in this book, you can thus benefit if you have any of the above.

In trying to understand why you are feeling sick, it is crucial to get to the root cause of your illness.

In my quest for health, I came across Functional Medicine. Functional Medicine as a practice, considers the myriad interactions among genetic, environmental, and lifestyle factors that can influence long-term health and complex, chronic disease. It addresses these factors holistically to optimise the functioning of your body, hence the term FUNCTIONAL MEDICINE.[1]

Throughout this document I have added the various sources. These are listed at the end of each section. This was done for three reasons:

1. so that you can see that the information provided is well researched,
2. to make it easier for you to read some more if you are interested, and
3. to give recognition to many experts out there who are willing to make such life changing information available for general consumption.

Let me get back to the point at hand. Functional Medicine asks how and why illness occurs and restores health by addressing the root causes of disease. My personal frustration with medical doctors is that they are trained to treat symptoms. They label you with a disease and send you away with a prescription focused at treating symptoms. **It is time that we all realise that by treating the root cause, we can regain our health!** Medical doctors do not get much training on nutrition. It is not their fault, but one can't ignore the root cause of illness and the benefit of nutrition. The functional medicine model highlights some root causes for chronic disease in the graphic below:

It is an approach to health care that conceptualizes health and illness as part of a continuum in which all components of the human biological system interact dynamically with the environment, producing patterns and effects that change over time.

Let's zoom in on some of these "hidden" root causes.

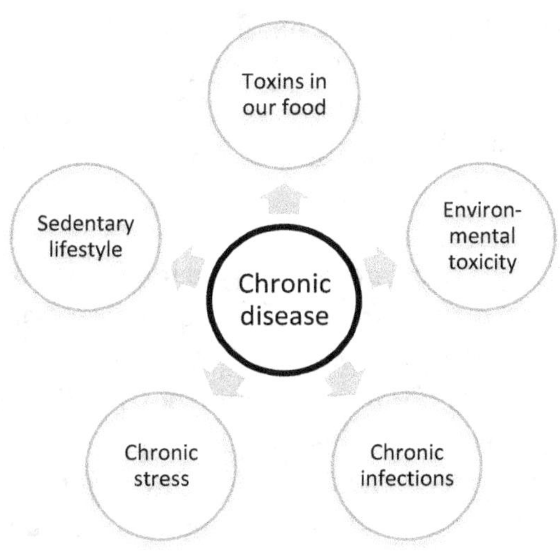

Toxins in our food

No matter what we eat, it is contaminated by hormones, pesticides, and all sorts of chemicals. Almost everything on our shelves are loaded with preservatives and/or are chemically modified. **Gluten being the biggest culprit**. Gluten harms our intestinal lining which allows impurities to enter our blood stream which wreaks havoc in our bodies. For anyone with severe body aches, allergies or skin issues, I would recommend you remove gluten from your diet for 3 weeks and see the impact for yourself.

Gut Permeability is also known as Leaky Gut. Dr Osborne indicates that Leaky Gut Syndrome typically develops slowly over time from the long-term exposure to inflammation within the digestive tract.[2]

As this inflammation continues over time, it first wears away the mucosal lining of the intestine which accounts for 80% of the immune system. Then as the damage continues, the inflammation begins to damage the cells of the intestines which has a two-pronged effect. It damages the cells that are responsible for secreting the enzymes that your body needs to properly digest your food. It also damages these cells in such a way that it causes them to lose their rigid structure. And instead of only allowing fully digested nutrients to pass through and enter your bloodstream, they begin to allow larger undigested food particles, toxins, bacteria, yeast, and pathogens direct access to your bloodstream.

Dr Tom O'Bryan says "typically the body cannot keep up with the task and a large portion of these foreign bodies will be absorbed into the tissues throughout the body, creating inflammation. This increases the levels of stress on your body. With your immune system focused on these enemies of the state, the smaller wars are going on unattended. These include filtering the blood, calming inflammation, fighting bacteria, regulating the workings of the gut, etc. This can lead to your body attacking itself, known as autoimmune disease". This could include any number of diseases including Chronic Fatigue, Multiple Sclerosis (MS), Irritable Bowel Syndrome (IBS), Ulcerative Colitis, Hashimotos, Lupus, Graves, Fibromyalgia and Type 1 Diabetes.[3]

Inflammation is a natural response by the body that is a part of the healing process. Due to the continuous strain we put our bodies under, the <u>*chronic*</u> *inflammation becomes a problem.*

Sue Ingebretson highlights the importance of removing gluten from your diet of you have any autoimmune disease or fibromyalgia. If you suffer from fibromyalgia, it is worth it to read the full article.[4]

Furthermore Dr Osborne quotes a study published in the medical journal *Nutrients* where it indicates that patients eating gluten show the following deficiencies: [5]

- ➢ 87.5% of patients diagnosed had at least 1 vitamin or mineral deficiency
- ➢ 53.8% were deficient in at least 2 nutrients
- ➢ 67% were deficient in the mineral zinc

- ➤ 46% were deficient in iron storage
- ➤ 20% were deficient in folate (vitamin B9)
- ➤ 32% were anaemic
- ➤ 19% were deficient in vitamin B12
- ➤ 14.5% were deficient in vitamin B6
- ➤ 7.5% were deficient in vitamin A
- ➤ 4.5% were deficient in vitamin D

It is quite scary that the damage of the gut lining caused by gluten as well as other factors, can directly lead to malabsorption of nutrients.

If you thus don't treat the root cause, you can drink as many supplements as you want, it won't absorb.[6]

Gluten (as defined by the FDA) generally refers to alpha gliadin gluten, which is gluten associated with wheat. Gluten is actually a family of proteins found in grains. All grain by definition has a different form of gluten.

Products labelled gluten free, made from corn, still contains corn gluten.

Here is a list of some grain products and the types of gluten they contain:

Wheat	-	Gliadin
Barley	-	Hordein
Oats	-	Avenin
Corn	-	Zien
Millet	-	Panicin
Rye	-	Secalinin
Rice	-	Orzenin

Sorgum   -   Kafirin

All the above can cause inflammation in the gut. When doing an elimination diet, all the above should be eliminated and gradually reintroduced to confirm sensitivity. From my personal experience, wheat, barley and rye are the worst.

Dr Osborne indicates that multiple sclerosis (MS) patients have been found to be sensitive to gluten. He also warns that many supplements contain corn filler, which contains gluten.[7]

What I appreciate most from Dr Osborne is that he supports all his statements by proper research.

He also highlights that most grains also contain glyphosate which is a pesticide that also damages the gut wall. This is another reason why grains are harmful to the gut.

If you wish to learn more about gluten and the dangers associated with gluten, refer to the following resources:

> Dr Tom O'Bryan http://thedr.com
> Dr Osborne https://drpeterosborne.com
> Dr Hyman http://drhyman.com
> Dr Axe https://draxe.com

Each of these authors publish various free resources, including YouTube videos on the dangers of gluten.

Other toxic culprits in our food are additives, MSG, colourants, flavourings and preservatives.

Dr Axe highlights the top 7 food additives that causes leaky gut: [8]

> "Meat glue" – otherwise known as microbial transglutaminase, this special enzyme serves to hold proteins together. It is commonly found in processed meats such as crab meat, fish balls and cold meats.

> Sugars are extremely common in all processed or modified foods.

> Sodium – high salt intake . Salt is hidden in all processed foods.

> Emulsifiers which are added to most processed foods.

> Organic acids such as alcohol – solvents in food and beverages.

> Gluten.

> Nanometric particles (flavourants and colourants) which improve the taste, colour and appearance of foods.

It is crucial to take a moment and ponder on this information!

Everything we buy off the shelf from a supermarket contains some or other form of food additives, colourants, flavourings and preservatives. All of which damage our gut lining and have a direct impact on our health!

What about MSG?

Processed foods are loaded with additives. Whole foods do not contain any additives. MSG (Monosodium glutamate), which is found in an estimated 80% of processed foods, sets off a variety of adverse reactions such as skin rashes, headaches, moodiness, irritability, IBS, heart palpitations, depression and more, depending on your tolerance.[9]

The extent to which you are affected by these problems depends on your ability to tolerate it, but regardless, eating foods laced with MSG is devastating to your organs.

In short, MSG has the ability to make people feel lousy in the short term and potentially very ill in the long-term.

Whole, unprocessed foods have the opposite effect.

Let's for a moment zoom into sugars. A major issue with sugar is that it has no nutritional value, and of course messes with your blood sugar.

WebMD indicates that sugar has multiple negative effects on the body. It affects:[10]

> ➢ The brain
> ➢ Your mood
> ➢ Your teeth
> ➢ Your joints
> ➢ Your skin
> ➢ Your liver
> ➢ Your heart
> ➢ Your pancreas
> ➢ Your kidneys
> ➢ Your body weight
> ➢ Your sexual health

Nutritionist Angelique Panagos says that "too much sugar can lead to insulin resistance, hormonal imbalance, blood sugar spikes, 'bad' bacteria and leaky gut syndrome, all of which are huge problems for our bodies." She highlights that eating a nutritious diet that is free from processed foods will help your body stay strong and **lessen inflammation**.[11]

Just as food from supermarkets is loaded with food additives etc, it is also loaded with sugar in order to improve the taste.

These excess refined sugars wreak havoc in your body!

Remember, everything with a "-ose" at the end of a word on food labels, contain sugar!

What about sweeteners?

Dr Axe says if you have not stopped using artificial sweeteners, start doing so immediately!! He indicates that research shows that frequent consumption of sweet tasting, non-caloric foods interferes with metabolic function. **Every single packaged food with a label that says sugar free, is likely to contain some form of artificial sweeteners.** He indicates that the 5 worst sweeteners are:[12]

1. Aspartame (Equal, Canderel)
2. Sucralose (Splenda)
3. Acesulfame K (ACE K, Equal Spoonful, Sweet One, Sweet 'n Safe, Canderel)[13]
4. Saccharin (Sweet 'N Low, Sweet Twin)
5. Xylitol, Sorbitol

Dr David Perlmutter in Regain Your Brain Docuseries says that **consuming diet drinks almost triples your risk for Alzheimers and doubles the risk for Diabetes.** It is best to avoid diet drinks and in particular diet fizzy drinks.

Look at the side effects of sugar as illustrated by Dr Osborne:[14]

(A big thank you to Dr Osborne who gave permission to use his graphic in this guide)

Shocking isn't it! And here you thought you were making a healthy choice by using artificial sugars!

Be wary of sweeteners in yogurts, sodas, chewing gum, sweetened cereals, bottled sauces, processed foods and almost all snack bars.

Healthy alternatives are maple syrup, coconut sugar, dates or raw honey. [15]

The Whole Daily reports that the top 7 triggers of autoimmune disease are:[16]

1.   Gluten
2.   Sugar
3.   Stress
4.   Dairy
5.   Hydrolysed Oils
6.   An unbalanced microbiome
7.   Environmental toxins

Let's consider dairy. Next to gluten, dairy is one of the most inflammatory foods. It is important to note that 50% of people who are gluten intolerant are also dairy intolerant. Dairy is also acid forming, and listen to this, it is full of hormones and antibiotics. Alternatives could be raw or organic milk or goats' milk. It is important though that you need to test your sensitivity using an elimination diet.[17]

> The Compounding Pharmacy of South Africa published some guidelines for an elimination diet... these can be downloaded from the following link: https://www.compounding.co.za/wp-content/uploads/2017/02/Comprehensive-Elimination-Diet.pdf.
>
> These will become very important throughout this programme.

Non-dairy sources of calcium include almonds, kale, oranges, collard greens, broccoli, figs, spinach, coconut milk and sesame seeds.

Toxins in our food cannot be taken lightly. A clean, whole food diet can transform your life! The choice is yours!

Another very toxic food source is hydrogenated oils and trans fats.

Autoimmune diseases are exacerbated by the consumption of hydrogenated vegetable oils or trans-fatty acids from the usage of hydrogenated oils.[18] Hydrogenated oils (those which are treated with hydrogen to increase shelf life) are known to increase inflammation in the body, leading to a weakened immune system.

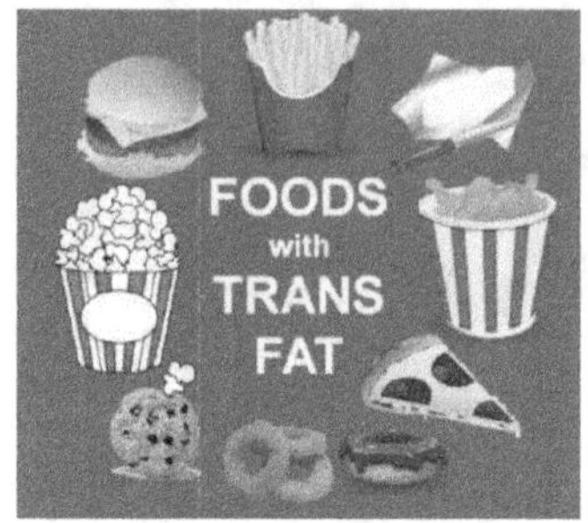

Some trans fats result when hydrogen is added to vegetable oil through the process of hydrogenation. Trans fats are more solid than oil and less likely to spoil, so the food has a longer shelf life.[19]

Trans fat tends to accumulate in the body and is not absorbed which tends to cause many complications like obesity and other medical conditions which may be potentially serious. Trans fat is mostly used in processed food.

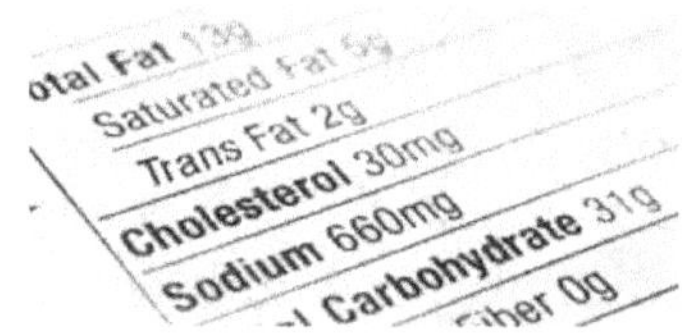

Toxins in our environment

Our environment is loaded with toxic substances. It starts with exhaust fumes, cleaning chemicals, perfumes, air fresheners, electromagnetic frequencies, bath soaps, non-stick pots and pans, plastic coffee lids (BPA), personal care products, pharmaceutical drugs, pesticides, phthalates, to mention but a few. They contain harmful chemicals which disrupt the endocrine system. **If we were only exposed to one or two our bodies would cope with it, but due to the magnitude of exposure, our bodies can't cope with the toxic load.**

Our daily accumulative toxic exposure is enormous and should not be underestimated.

Dr Axe highlights the top 10 toxic household items (Section 17 unpacks these in great detail):

1. Bleach[20]
2. Anti-bacterial chemicals (e.g. water free hand cleaners)

3. Scented candles and air fresheners
4. Talcum baby powder
5. Dry cleaning chemicals
6. Vinyl flooring / curtains
7. Volatile Compounds (VOC's) contained in, for example, laundry detergents
8. Flame retardants found in, for example, mattresses[21]
9. Pesticides
10. Non-stick pans

Without us even realising, we are exposing our bodies to severe toxic loads. If we were only exposed to one or two of these our bodies would have been able to cope with the load. **The challenge is that everything we eat, everything we are exposed to in our households, and everything we use for personal care is toxic.** Our bodies can only take so much. Realistically we could never remove all toxins from our environment. And as such our bodies have been masterfully designed to cope with toxins.

The challenge is the excessive load. We should all, within our means, start at one point and slowly remove the big culprits from our lives. As you do this, you will quickly see an improvement in your heath!

In section 17 on environmental toxins, we will explore these environmental toxins in more detail and look at healthy alternatives.

Dr Tom O'Bryan quotes shocking statistics. He indicates that in a study over 38 years, they found a sperm reduction of 59 % across the board. Once 72% is reached, the extinction of humankind is in question. He emphasises that the toxins in our environment and food all contribute to such statistics.[22]

Wendy Myers is a nutritionist who specialises in heavy metal detoxification. She highlights the most common heavy metals we are exposed to on a daily basis:[23]

- ➤ Aluminium - in the air, deodorants and vaccines
- ➤ Thallium – petroleum
- ➤ Cesium – nuclear disasters
- ➤ Arsenic – common in rice, chicken, eggs
- ➤ Tin – Amalgam fillings

Dr Hyman highlights the risk of mercury poisoning. Two sources can include silver fillings in your teeth and tuna.

Wendy Myers says that metal toxicity can have a major impact on energy levels.

> Supplements such as binders, minerals, magnesium and Epsom salt bath salts can also help. Coffee enemas is also useful. Exercise can help, but in the event of major heavy metal toxicity, low impact exercises are better such as yoga, walking or swimming.
> As for diet, animal protein is crucial for detoxification. About 15% of your intake should be protein. Vegans do have challenges with detoxification. Drinking enough water is crucial.
> **If detoxification is happening too fast, it can create severe symptoms. In which case a slower detox is required.**

I have been on the receiving end of detoxing too fast. I bought an online detox programme from a reputable supplier. It basically was a two-week no meat, only fruit and veggies diet. At the time I was extremely toxic. I could not even go for a massage without being in agony during the massage and very sick after. This detox amplified all my symptoms. I urge you not to move too fast with a detox if your body is severely inflamed. Rather make lifestyle changes that will naturally clean out your body. In this programme, all such strategies will be explored.

If you think you may have heavy metal toxicity, it's best to work with a functional health practitioner, homeopath or an integrative health practitioner. DO NOT GO AT IT ALONE!

What I love about Wendy Myers is that she also emphasises that detoxification is a lifestyle. Thus, changing your lifestyle such that you prevent toxifying your body and supporting your body on a continuous basis to detoxify.

Dr Ben Johnson highlights that toxins, pathogens (a bacterium, virus, or other microorganism that can cause disease) and emotions are our primary causes of disease. He specialises in skin conditions and says that he very early in his career realised that the root causes of skin conditions are not on the surface, but rather inside the body and more particularly in the gut.[24]

Sedentary lifestyle

In this information age, we are either stuck in traffic or stuck behind our computers. We do not walk enough, nor move our bodies enough. We must get moving!

Our heart is the power behind your cardiovascular circulatory system, pumping blood through your blood vessels, supplying every part of your body with the oxygen and nutrients it needs for proper functioning. With poor circulation, not only is your blood flow impaired, compromising that blood supply, but your heart is unduly taxed. Both have negative consequences and can lead to a variety of health problems.

"Poor circulation can lead directly to heart attack, stroke, eye disease, kidney disease, and claudication (leg muscle pain or weakness that comes and goes after an activity like walking)," says Dr. David Katz, Associate Professor in Public Health Practice at the Yale University School of Public Health and director of the Integrative Medicine Center in Derby, CT. "But poor circulation also plays a role in almost every disease, from dementia to diabetes, influenza to cirrhosis."[25]

Your lymphatic circulatory system works directly with your cardiovascular circulatory system to keep blood and lymphatic fluid levels in balance and flush toxins out of the body. It also carries immune cells throughout the body to help defend against infections.

But your lymphatic system isn't lucky enough to have a powerful organ like the heart to keep fluid flowing. "The lymph system is stimulated by gravity, muscle contraction (exercise), hydrotherapy (alternating hot and cold water on the skin), breathing, lymph drainage therapy, and massage," says Harper (MediSpa).

If your lymphatic circulation slows or stagnates, toxins will accumulate and immune cells won't be delivered to the areas of the body where they're needed, causing a variety of ailments, the very least of which are aches, pains, and swelling (lymph edema).

This can also cause deterioration of your thymus gland, tonsils, and spleen which are key components of your immune system. This will weaken your body's ability to fight infection and disease.

> Here are some activities that improve circulation:
> 1. Drinking lots of water
> 2. Regular exercise or movement
> 3. Healthy eating habits

It is crucial for your health to start moving and get the blood flowing in your veins.

Chronic stress

Stress is a state of mental or emotional strain or tension resulting from adverse or demanding circumstances. It must be seen in relation to the demands you are faced with.

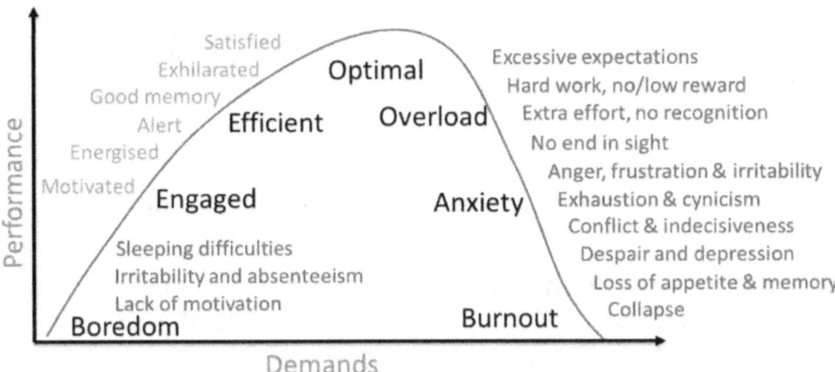

Demands directly impact your performance and if the demands are too many or too intense for too long, it can lead to burnout.

All types of stress are not by default bad! Stress can also enhance performance. Positive stress is referred to as eustress, while negative stress is referred to as distress. It is very interesting that if the demands in your life and in the workplace, are too low, it also causes distress.

As can be seen in the Burnout Curve above, if you are underutilised and not exposed to demands in line with your abilities, you will be bored, which will lead to sleeping difficulties, irritability, absenteeism and lack of motivation. But if you are exposed to demands aligned with your abilities and capacity, you will be engaged, efficient and function optimally at the top of the curve. Then you will feel motivated, energised and alert, display good memory and feel exhilarated and satisfied. Once the demands exceed that optimal level, and the pressure becomes too much, overload and anxiety set in, which ultimately lead to burnout. In this process, you are exposed to excessive expectations and demands, either from others or yourself.

You will put in a lot of effort but will not feel that you are getting the reward for your hard work. Then you will try even harder and work even longer hours, which will exacerbate the feeling that you are not recognised for what you do. It will start to feel that there is no end in sight, which will culminate in major frustration, irritability and anger. You will start to feel exhausted and cynical. As the pressure mounts, you will become indecisive and experience conflict in relationships. Despair, depression and loss of appetite will set in. In some cases, it culminates in an increased appetite. You will start to forget even the smallest little detail. You will walk into a room to get something and will get there not knowing what you were looking for. And before you know it, you will collapse. Collapse is the final stage of burnout.

The adrenal glands are two glands that sit on top of your kidneys. They are made up of two distinct parts.[26]

The adrenal cortex which is the outer part of the gland, produces hormones that are vital to life, such as cortisol. These help regulate metabolism and help your body respond to stress. It also produces aldosterone, which helps control blood pressure.

The adrenal medulla is the inner part of the gland. The adrenal medulla produces nonessential hormones, such as adrenaline. Adrenaline is not essential to life, but helps your body react to stress.

Cortisol plays a key role in burnout. It is produced in the cortex of the adrenal glands and is transported around your body via the bloodstream. When your adrenal glands are overworked and exhausted, the mechanisms that control this process can very quickly become dysregulated. This can result in erratic spikes of cortisol at inappropriate times. If this continues to happen more and more frequently, it will eventually lead to burnout.

Shirra Moch is a lecturer in the Department of Pharmacy, Pharmacology and Health Sciences at the University of the Witwatersrand in Johannesburg, South Africa. The focus of her research is stress. Moch and her colleagues conducted a study on 16 people who suffered a stress burnout so severe that they had to be hospitalised. She reported that they mostly spent the day in bed, crying. Normally, when peoples' bodies are stressed by an illness, or their minds are stressed by external circumstances or even an argument with a spouse, the body secretes the hormone cortisol. This hormone helps the body fight off disease. Many overstressed people have too much cortisol, but the people Moch studied had low cortisol levels.[27]

Moch's patients were given intensive stress management therapy while they were in hospital, which included medication and courses in meditation, breathing, exercise and nutrition. They also saw a social worker who taught them to handle stressful situations and a psychiatrist who gave them talk therapy. They participated in this programme all day for about five days while in hospital and then half days for a short time after they were discharged. Afterwards, they came in for monthly follow-up sessions.

The intense stress management worked only up to a point. The people with burnout did start to feel better and were able to go back to work and live normal lives. However, their cortisol levels remained low, even after five months. This means they remained more susceptible to diseases like colds and flu and were more likely to have another burnout episode if they didn't adhere to the stress management changes they were taught.

Moch presented these findings at the 32nd Annual Meeting of the International Society of Psychoneuroendocrinology. Moch stated: "When they feel well, they start to backslide right away (on the stress management programme), it's only when they start to feel sick again that they think, 'oh yes, I have to do all this stuff again!' We're trying to educate them that this is lifestyle change."

Developing lifestyle habits that support proactive stress management is key to good health.

Electro Magnetic Frequencies (EMF)

EMF is starting to get the attention it deserves. Research has now found that EMF can cause DNA damage. People all over the world are starting to experience various symptoms that cannot be explained. This includes skin problems, itchiness, light sensitivity, fatigue, blood pressure, headaches, joint and muscle pain and dizziness.[28] Electronics that emit EMF include cell phones, smart meters, cordless phones, circuit breaker panels, microwaves, cell phone towers, WiFi etc.

This topic will be addressed in more detail in Section 17 as part of environmental toxins.

Should you experience any unexplained symptoms, put you WiFi on a timer for a start, or consider wiring your computer so that you can switch the WiFi off. Do not use your cell phone next to your ear, use an ear phone or the speaker phone. And do NOT sleep with your phone next to your bed.

Chronic infections

Infections are common throughout our lifetime, but rarely do they lead to an autoimmune disorder. By the time you are 20 years old, it's likely that you've been exposed to or had a few infections.

Scientists believe that a variety of factors must usually be present for an infection to result in an autoimmune condition, including a genetic predisposition and other lifestyle factors, including stress, poor diet, poor sleep and leaky gut.

According to many healthcare practitioners who treat autoimmune conditions, if patients don't get better after addressing food triggers and correcting nutrient deficiencies, it's time to dig deeper and test for hidden infections.[29]

The Healing is Freedom website provides a great summary of common infections linked to specific autoimmune disorders *(note that this list is not comprehensive):*

Autoimmune Disorder	Commonly Linked Infection
Multiple sclerosis (MS)	Human herpesvirus 6 (HHV-6), Epstein-Barr virus (EBV aka herpesvirus 4), Rubella, influenza virus, and Human Papilloma Virus (HPV), Chlamydia, Borrelia burgdorferi, and measles virus
Type 1 diabetes	Coxsackievirus B4, cytomegalovirus (CMV), mumps virus, and rubella virus
Rheumatoid arthritis (RA)	EBV, hepatitis C virus, E-coli bacteria, Citrobacter, Klebsiella, Proteus, Parvovirus, Mycoplasma infection
Sjogren's Syndrome	EBV
Systemic lupus erythematosus (SLE)	EBV
Myocarditis	CB3, CMV, Chlamydia
Hashimoto's thyroiditis & Graves	Porphyromonas Yersinia, EBV
Myasthenia gravis	Hepatitis C virus (HCV), herpes simplex virus
Guillain-Barré syndrome	EBV, CMV, Campylobacter bacteria
Autoimmune urticaria, psoriasis, alopecia areata and Schoenlein-Henoch purpura	Helicobacter pylori (H. pylori)
Celiac Disease, Irritable Bowel Syndrome (IBS), Inflammatory Bowel Disease (IBD), Crohn's Disease	Small Intestinal Bacterial Overgrowth (SIBO)

    Your Greatest Wealth is your Health   33

> The first step in treating an autoimmune disease is lifestyle changes with an emphasis on eating habits, exercise and sleeping habits.
> Should a patient not respond well to these, it is advised that they engage a functional medicine practitioner to confirm if they do not suffer from a chronic infection.

Work with your functional medicine practitioner to identify and treat any underlying infections. Do not go at it alone.

By now you should have a real appreciation for why so many of us are walking around not feeling well. Hang in there, it is not all gloom and doom. I know you may feel a bit overwhelmed now. By the end of this book you will have all the tools to take charge of your health.

What is the end result of all these triggers discussed above? Let's explore in the next section.

Sources of References in Section 2

1.   https://p.widencdn.net/xazlwe/Intro_Functional_Medicine

2.   https://www.glutenfreesociety.org/leaky-gut-week

3.   http://thedr.com

4.   http://www.prohealth.com/library/showarticle.cfm?libid=18639

5.   https://www.glutenfreesociety.org/leaky-gut-week

6.   **Source:** Wierdsma NJ, van Bokhorst-de van der Schueren MA, Berkenpas M, et al. Vitamin and mineral deficiencies are highly prevalent in newly diagnosed celiac disease patients. Nutrients. 2013 Sep 30;5(10):3975-92. doi: 10.3390/nu5103975.

7.   https://www.youtube.com/watch?v=WEsoHNZqvto&inf_contact_key =b1b2351f468a857ccd46eba2683cba150b5808664e0b96bc362adcecb7 8c0a01

8.   https://draxe.com/7-food-additives-that-trigger-leaky-gut/

9.   https://www.bewell.com/blog/no-more-msg-the-dangerous-food-additive-you-must-live-without/

10. https://www.webmd.com/diet/features/how-sugar-affects-your-body

11. https://iquitsugar.com/sugar-autoimmune-disease/

12. https://draxe.com/artificial-sweeteners/

13. https://regainyourbrain.awakeningfromalzheimers.com/

14. https://drpeterosborne.com/artificial-sweeteners-toxic-side-effects/

15. http://www.greenmedinfo.com/blog/why-you-should-ditch-sugar-favor-honey

16. http://thewholedaily.com.au/health/top-7-triggers-auto-immune-disease/

17. https://www.mindbodygreen.com/0-8646/the-dangers-of-dairy.html

18. http://thewholedaily.com.au/health/top-7-triggers-auto-immune-disease/

19. https://allontario.ca/everything-about-trans-fats/

20. https://www.youtube.com/watch?v=qrBm62PBuWQ&feature=em-subs_digest

21. http://www.greenmedinfo.com/blog/truth-about-toxic-mattresses

22. http://theheavymetalssummit.com/expert/tom-obryan/

23. http://theheavymetalssummit.com/expert/wendy-myers/

24. http://theheavymetalssummit.com/expert/ben-johnson/

25. https://www.gaiam.com/blogs/discover/6-ways-to-boost-circulation-for-detoxing-and-immunity

26. https://www.endocrineweb.com/endrocronology/overview-adrenal-glands

27. http://www.webmd.com/balance/stress-management/news/20010815/stressed-out-dont-let-become-burnout

28. https://hingetee.ee/meedia/2018/04/emf_protection_free_report.pdf

29. http://www.healingisfreedom.com/science/top-5-autoimmune-triggers-infections/

Section 3

Leaky Gut or Gut Permeability

THE RESULT - POOR GUT HEALTH

What is gut permeability? And why does it matter?

The father of modern medicine, Hippocrates, said, "All disease begins in the gut." Gut Permeability, Intestinal Permeability or Leaky Gut refers to damage of the gut lining which allows material passing from inside the gastrointestinal tract through the cells lining the gut wall, into the rest of the body, through the blood stream.

Dr Osborne says that "one of the most common symptoms associated with Leaky Gut Syndrome is food allergies. As undigested food particles begin passing freely through the intestinal lining, the remaining 20% of the immune system is left to clean up the mess. So, it begins to target the foods that you eat as the problem, and when your immune system builds up antigens against these foods then they present themselves to you as food allergies. Because 80% of the immune system exists within that mucosal barrier that lines a healthy digestive tract, your immune system has already taken a beating in this Leaky Gut process.[1]

Over time, this continuous damage takes its toll leaving you susceptible to chronic infections, chronic Candida (yeast) symptoms and eventually autoimmune conditions such as arthritis, eczema, and psoriasis"

Dr Partha Nandi, in the Candida Summit hosted by Evan Brand, emphasises the link between candida and leaky gut, and subsequently inflammation, which then translates into allergies and skin disorders, and a host of other symptoms. He says to avoid fast foods and processed foods, and to reduce stressors in your life. He highly recommends eating whole foods.[2]

Symptoms of leaky gut

According to Dr Axe there are 7 Leaky Gut symptoms and signs namely: [3]

1. Food sensitivities
2. Inflammatory bowel disease
3. Autoimmune disease
4. Thyroid problems
5. Nutrient malabsorption
6. Inflammatory skin conditions
7. Mood issues and autism

Dr Tom O'Bryan states that the impact of leaky gut is on the weak link in your chain. In other words, if your body is a chain, all of us have a weak link. That could be your skin, heart, stomach, brain and so forth. Some common symptoms listed by Dr O'Bryan are:[4]

1. Multiple food sensitivities
2. Nutritional deficiencies
3. Chronic diarrhoea and constipation
4. Skin rashes
5. Headaches
6. Brain fog
7. Memory loss
8. Excessive fatigue
9. Yeast (Candida) and bacterial overgrowth (SIBO)

According to Dr O'Bryan, dietary issues that could contribute to leaky gut are high intake of **refined sugars, processed foods, food**

additives, preservatives, refined flours and artificial flavourings.

Are you starting to see a pattern? The only answer is organic whole foods!

Dr O'Bryan agrees with Dr Osborne in that chronic stress suppresses the immune system which doesn't allow it to do its job properly and it gets overrun with pathogens very quickly. This leads to increased inflammation in the intestines and increased permeability to the gut lining.[5]

Chronic stress, meaning all stress that is put on the body. It includes emotional stress, poor food choice stress and environmental toxin stress.

He indicates that any type of inflammation in the gut can cause leaky gut. **Some reasons for inflammation are low stomach acid, yeast of bacterial overgrowth (Candida / SIBO), infections, parasites and excessive environmental toxins.** He also highlights that medications, including aspirin, acetaminophen and ibuprofen irritate the intestinal lining and decreases the mucosal levels, which are the first line of defence in the intestines.

Did you get that? The medicines you take that are supposed to treat your symptoms could cause your symptoms!

Do not stop taking any prescribed medicines without talking to your functional medicine practitioner.

Dr O'Bryan refers to work done by Dr Fassano that indicates that Gluten and Lipopolysaccharides (LPS) are the main triggers for intestinal permeability. LPS is made of fats (lipids) and sugar. This compound is both structural and protective to normally benign bacteria. However, when released into the bloodstream, LPS is a potent endotoxin (coming from within) and drives a sudden and acute inflammatory reaction.[6]

Dr Michael Klaper emphasises that by what we eat, drink and medicine we take, we kill off the good bacteria in our bodies which causes dysbiosis. Check out the link at the end of this section for a video if you are interested in more information. [7]

Natalie Cruttenden indicates that Small Intestinal Bowel Overgrowth (SIBO) could be a major issue in the treatment of gut issues.[8] SIBO happens when bacteria that belong in the large intestine move up into the small intestine. She highlights that a major symptom of SIBO is food sensitivities. It would also cause people to react to certain foods, and not always the same foods. Other symptoms are bloating, gas, constipation, diarrhoea, fatigue and brain fog. Dr Nirala Jacobi says bloating directly after meals is a major symptom.[9]

Treatment depends on the type of gas one's body releases. If Hydrogen gas, she typically recommends Refaximin, clove and oregano. In the case of Methane gas, she recommends garlic and neem.

> She says that proteins and fats are safe for people with SIBO. Carbohydrates pose a problem as bacteria thrive on carbs. She says two thirds of your plate should be vegetables and a third protein with added healthy fats.

It is CRUCIAL to work with a functional medical practitioner to rule out and treat SIBO.

Medicine and the gut

Dr Osborne emphasises that the average adult over age 35 is on 3 or more medications. Some of the most common ones include drugs for pain, heartburn, depression, thyroid disease, antibiotics, cholesterol, and high blood pressure.[10] I am sure you can all relate.

Seeing that these medicines contribute to leaky gut, the consequence of these medications can contribute to the loss of iron, magnesium, calcium, zinc, potassium, vitamin B12, biotin, vitamin K, vitamin C, vitamin B1, and folate.

The sad irony is that doctors give the drugs to "treat" disease, but by "treating" patients this way, nutritional loss is the end result.[11] Many of the symptoms being medicated are the same symptoms caused by the nutritional loss. He for instance says that high blood pressure drugs cause magnesium loss, and magnesium loss causes high blood pressure. How do you escape this vicious cycle?

> The answer is – KNOWLEDGE. Making sure your doctor tests for vitamin and mineral deficiencies is an essential first step. Nutritional supplementation while on these medications is also a priority, but beware that many vitamins contain gluten.
>
> TREAT THE ROOT CAUSE - Heal your leaky gut.

Don't flush your money and health down the toilet. A recent study investigated over the counter vitamin and mineral supplements for the presence of gluten, and the results were alarming for those who are trying to follow a gluten free diet and maintain a healthy lifestyle through the use of multi-vitamins, probiotics, etc.[12] *Almost 24% of the products tested had enough gluten in them to create inflammatory damage.*

Read the labels of your medication before buying or using them.

Causes of leaky gut

Let's understand why we get leaky gut. Even though we have touched on this before, I would like to explore it some more. This is a key step in your journey.

According to Anthony Haynes and Antoinette Savill (The Food Intolerance Bible) the following are the main causes of leaky gut:[13]

Take a few minutes and read these carefully!!

1. **Eating foods to which you have an intolerance**

   It is also known as allergic gastroenteropathy. Where food intolerances exist, leaky gut follows. It lowers Secretary IgA which leads to emotional frustration and leaky gut.

2. **Alcohol**

   Alcohol creates a deficiency in N-Acetyl-Glucosamine (NAG), a building block for the cells in the intestine.

3. **Antibiotics**

   Antibiotics inhibit friendly bacteria in the gut that plays a key role in maintaining the tummy wall.

4. **Non-steroidal anti-inflammatory drugs (NSAIDs)**

   NSAIDs such as ibuprofen and aspirin have the following impact:

   a) They create a deficiency in N-Acetyl-Glucosamine (NAG)

   b) They interrupt the secretion of protective substances called prostaglandins

   c) They bind to and prevent the function of the most abundant protective phospholipid that lines the intestinal wall lining.

5. **Corticosteroids** – such as prednisone, cortisone and other steroid medication affects the rate at which the intestinal lining heals itself.

6. Eating too much of the same foods and eating them too often

Eating the same foods too often leads to lack of nutrients required for optimal gut health.

7. Sugar

Refined sugar has no nutritional value. Sugar weakens the immune system for a number of hours after being consumed.

8. Amino Acid deficiency

Amino acids are required to nourish the intestinal lining. L-Glutamine and N-Acetyl-Glucosamine are most important.

9. Zinc and or Vitamin A deficiency

Zinc is vital for growth and healing in the body. Vitamin A is needed for epithelial growth and repair (tissue that lines the cavities and surfaces of body's organs).

10. Digestive tract infections

Unwanted, unfriendly bacteria can disrupt normal intestinal ecology and permeability. Parasites and yeast overgrowth can also damage the intestinal lining.

11. Stress

Stress lowers our intestinal defences and make us prone to inflammatory reactions. It negatively impacts digestion.

12. Poor digestion

Lack of digestive enzymes, also called stomach acids, lead to inflammation which leads to leaky gut. Chewing food well is very important.

13. Inflammatory bowel disease

Chron's, ulcerative colitis and celiac can all lead to leaky gut. It is possible that leaky gut could also be the cause of inflammatory bowel disease.[14]

14. Antacids and proton pump inhibitors (PPIs)

Long term use of antacids and PPIs leads to leaky gut. In an emergency it can save your life, but it is not designed for long term chronic use.

Have you perhaps identified one or more of your issues?

Addressing a leaky gut

Dr Kelly Ann explains the process as follows:[15]

1. First your gut flora gets out of balance.

Did you ever get a prescription for an antibiotic and find yourself running to the bathroom every few hours? That's because in addition to killing off bad bacteria, antibiotics kill off trillions of good bacteria. Without those beneficial bacteria, bad bacteria and fungi that are resistant to an antibiotic can take over and inflame your gut. Getting your gut bacteria out of balance.

While antibiotics are big offenders when it comes to unbalancing gut flora, there are other culprits as well such as stress, lack of sleep, lack of exercise, wrong diet and antacids. Antacids are over-the-counter medications that help neutralize stomach acid.

The biggest culprit of all is a sugary, high-starch diet.

2. Secondly your gut biochemistry changes.

When your good bacteria reduce relative to the bad bacteria, they can't keep your digestion up to speed. You get fewer nutrients like zinc, vitamin C, and omega-3 fatty acids, which feed your skin cells (and all cells) and keep them young and vibrant.

When good flora get too depleted, they can't efficiently synthesize hormones and certain vitamins. The result is that your skin gets dry, wrinkly, and develops a dull greyish look as your levels of anti-aging hormones, B vitamins, and vitamin K drop.

3. Your Peyer's patches come under attack.

When bad flora takes over your gut, they produce toxins that inflame your Peyer's patches. Peyer's patches are small masses of lymphatic tissue found throughout the ileum region of the small intestine. They form an important part of the immune system by monitoring intestinal bacteria populations and preventing the growth of pathogenic bacteria in the intestines.[16]

These patches grow weak, allowing toxins to stream in and causing leaky gut. As your gut barrier becomes more and more permeable, toxins that should stay in your intestines escape into your bloodstream.

Dr Kelly Ann indicates that some of the steps you can take are:

- Banish sugar, flour, and other high-carb foods from your diet. Bad bacteria thrive on these foods and your skin hates them. She says that a leading dermatology journal recently branded carbs as the "main culprit" in acne. Centre your diet around low-carb proteins, veggies, and healthy fats, and banish donuts and sugared cereal from your diet.

- Repopulate your good flora. Eat fermented foods like sauerkraut, kefir, and yogurt, which recharge your gut with helpful bacteria. Take a high-quality probiotic supplement daily. And eat lots of veggies, which feed your good bacteria the nutrients they need.

- Get more exercise. She says that researchers in Ireland reported that exercise increases the diversity of bacteria in the gut. In particular, the exercisers they studied had higher levels of a bacterium called Akkermansiaceae, which lowers inflammation. As a bonus, it also protects against obesity.

- De-stress. Stress kills off good gut bacteria and causes potentially harmful ones to multiply. To fight stress, deploy stress management techniques such as yoga, take a walk in nature, and other activities you find relaxing every day.

- Take antibiotics only if you need them. These drugs won't do you any good if you have a virus, and the damage they do to your gut flora is long-lasting. If you do need to take them, load up on prebiotics and probiotics afterward, and enjoy fermented foods.

In addition to damaging your internal organs, these toxins wreak havoc on your skin. They send your immune system into wild overdrive, causing rashes and dermatitis. They break down your skin's natural defences, leading to acne. And they create body-wide inflammation, turning your skin red, puffy, and spotty.

Food intolerances and gut permeability

Food intolerances can wreak havoc in your body. They are typically a sign that your tummy wall is not in the state it should be. According to Anthony Haynes and Antoinette Saville (The Food Intolerance

Bible, 2005) it is crucial to understand why we have food intolerances.[17]

Reasons could include:

1. Eating too much of the same food too often
2. Food additives, preservatives, colouring agents and flavour enhancers
3. Eating too quickly
4. Maldigestion (low stomach acid levels of pancreatic enzymes)
5. Imbalanced intestinal ecology: an overgrowth of yeast, bacteria or parasites
6. Prescription or over the counter medicine
7. Weak intestinal immunity
8. Excess stress

It is interesting that all the above could lead to leaky gut. Hence it is vital to address these factors.

Dr Hyman, in his Broken Brain Docuseries, indicates that food intolerances or allergies fit into two categories.[18] One is when you immediately react to a given food. A great example is nut allergies. People with severe nut allergies immediately feel their throats close up. The second type is where you have a delayed response. A person may eat gluten and only experience a mood swing or headache hours or a day or two later. These are more difficult to pinpoint. Foods that typically fit into this category are gluten, dairy and food additives, preservatives, colouring agents and flavour enhancers.

The content of the Broken Brain series are as follows:
1. The Broken Brain Epidemic / My Story
2. Gut Brain Connection: Getting to The Root of a Broken Brain
3. Losing Your Mind (Alzheimer's, Dementia and MS)

4. ADHD and Autism
5. Depression & Anxiety
6. Traumatic Brain Injury: Accidents, Sports and More
7. Seven Steps to An UltraMind (Part 1)
8. Seven Steps to An UltraMind (Part 2)

It is amazing that in this docuseries, leaky gut is directly linked to brain / neurological disorders. And even more amazing, is that through changing eating habits and reducing environmental toxins, patients either get much better or even reverse their illnesses.

The best way to confirm food intolerances are to avoid these foods for two weeks and then to reintroduce them one at a time. The resultant effects should be more noticeable.

The reason why food intolerances are so important when you follow this programme, is that you must realise that some food intolerances are common to most people such as gluten, dairy and food additives, preservatives, colouring agents and flavour enhancers. Other food intolerances greatly depend on the person.

So even though certain foods may be really good for you, if you have an intolerance, it could harm your body.

Jordan Reasoner is a health engineer and author. He says that **if you're having sensitivities to more than a dozen different foods, you likely have leaky gut.**[19]

The good news is that as you heal your leaky gut, you can gradually reintroduce these foods and there is a high likelihood that you could eat these again and that your intolerance would have magically disappeared. But should you re-introduce foods and have any symptom, it is best to avoid such foods.

     Your Greatest Wealth is your Health   **47**

Hopefully you now have an appreciation of just how important it is for ALL OF US to treat ourselves for leaky gut. Chances are that most of us have leaky gut as a result of the various toxic foods and environmental toxins we are exposed to on a daily basis. Let's come to grips what the sad outcome is of having leaky gut. Not only can it lead to autoimmune disorders, it can also lead to mood disorders, stubborn belly fat, brain degeneration, skin disorders and hormone imbalances.

Sources of References in Section 3

1. https://www.glutenfreesociety.org/leaky-gut-week/
2. https://candidasummit.com/expert/partha-nandi/
3. https://draxe.com/7-signs-symptoms-you-have-leaky-gut/)
4. http://be-gluten-free.com/leaky-gut-affecting-health/
5. http://be-gluten-free.com/leaky-gut-affecting-health/
6. http://realfoodcon.com/dr-tom-obryan/
7. https://www.youtube.com/watch?v=QRDoqS6QHQw&feature=em
8. https://healthygutexperts.com/day-5/natalie-cruttenden/
9. https://healthygutexperts.com/day-5/dr-nirala-jacobi/
10. https://www.glutenfreesociety.org/leaky-gut-week/
11. https://healthygutexperts.com/day-5/dr-nirala-jacobi/
12. Pelton R, LaValle J, Hawkins EB, Krinsky DL. The Drug-Induced Nutrient Depletion Handbook. Lexi-Comp, Inc.
13. Anthony Haynes and Antoinette Savill - The Food Intolerance Bible
14. https://lectinfreemama.com/2017/07/09/blocking-stomach-acid/
15. https://www.drkellyann.com/about-dr-kellyann/
16. https://www.drkellyann.com/about-dr-kellyann/
17. Anthony Haynes and Antoinette Savill - The Food Intolerance Bible
18. https://brokenbrain.com/
19. https://scdlifestyle.com/2010/03/the-scd-diet-and-leaky-gut-syndrome/

Section 4

Autoimmune disease, including diabetes

THE NEXT LOGICAL STEP AFTER LEAKY GUT: AUTOIMMUNE DISEASE

The body attacking itself

According to Dr Tom O'Bryan, autoimmune disease is the number three cause of becoming sick or dying. Dr O'Bryan indicates that autoimmune diseases start early in life with a slow progression, which increases as you grow older. You may now think back and realise that you have had vague symptoms for many years. That is because it took many years to evolve to the state where it is today.[1]

Let's take a minute to understand the immune system. Reality is that we all have multiple viruses, fungi, bacteria and other pathogens in our bodies. A healthy immune system can handle these. It is called the immune response.[2]

The immune system protects the body from harmful influences in the environment. We have covered all these up to this point in the guide. **The immune response is the body's way to protect itself against viruses, bacteria or any foreign invaders or organisms. When the immune system is weak or suppressed, this protection is compromised.**

We all have this innate immunity which we are born with. Our first line of defence against germs include our skin, as well as the lining of our respiratory and digestive tract. If a virus or microbe gets past this wall, our white blood cells launch a defensive attack. This is called our Cellular immunity. It works mainly through phagocytosis (swallowing up the organism). Most of the time the white blood cells can do the job. If the white cells fail, our Humoral immunity is called into action. Our Humoral immunity then launches our chemical defence mechanism viz. our Th1 and Th2 defence mechanism. The Th1 mechanism is similar to hand-to-hand combat while the Th2 is similar to chemical warfare. Collectively these defence mechanisms keep us safe. The problem arises when these defence mechanisms get hyper stimulated and run into overdrive. They then cause autoimmune diseases. They can then turn the body against itself. The antibodies then attack body tissue instead of foreign invaders.[3]

According to Mickey Trescott the list below shows the conditions that are most commonly associated with a Th1 or Th2 dominant state.[4]

TH1 dominant conditions	TH2 dominant conditions
Type I diabetes	Lupus
Multiple sclerosis	Allergic Dermatitis
Hashimoto's Thyroiditis	Scleroderma
Graves Disease	Atopic Eczema
Crohn's Disease	Sinusitis
Psoriasis	Inflammatory Bowel Disease
Sjoren's Syndrome	Asthma
Celiac Disease	Allergies
Lichen Planus	Cancer
Rheumatoid Arthritis	Ulcerative Colitis
Chronic viral infections	Multiple chemical sensitivity

Dr O'Bryan says 5 in 7 of people have antibodies against some tissue in their bodies. He indicates that research has shown that autoimmune disease starts at least 9-10 years before they are diagnosed.[5]

Dr O'Bryan says every degenerative disease is a disease of inflammation in the cells. First priority is to reduce inflammation.

In other words, the cells are on fire. The long and the short is, put the fire out. Then you can slow down or arrest the autoimmune disease. He says" stop throwing gasoline on the fire".

The biggest awareness you can come to, is **"Everything we eat and drink is either inflammatory of anti-inflammatory"**. The inflammatory foods will impact the weak link in your body. Whatever that may be. This is a very important point to understand to get you closer to your healing! **Removing the root cause of your inflammation and bombarding your body with anti-inflammatory foods will become very important going forward.**

Paula Owens indicates that the root causes of autoimmune diseases are a genetic susceptibility, toxic chemical exposure and leaky gut. (And poor food choices lead to leaky gut!)[6]

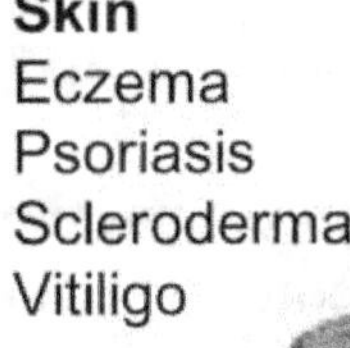

From the graphic it becomes evident that if you have any of the diseases listed, lifestyle changes aimed at supporting your microbiome or healing your leaky gut will greatly enhance your health!

Dr Tom O'Bryan says that molecular mimicry is a major cause of autoimmune disease. He uses the example of gluten. The body releases anti-bodies to protect itself. It confuses gluten for proteins in the body by mimicking those proteins. In my case gluten mimics my thyroid. When I eat gluten, my immune system does not recognise that it is gluten and mistakes the gluten for my thyroid and ends up attacking both.

Leaky gut and mitochondrial disfunction

Research by Clark and Mach shows a bidirectional interaction between mitochondria and microbiota (the condition of your gut). [7] This means that your gut health affects your mitochondria.

Mitochondria are components within our cells from which we derive 90% of our energy. If your mitochondria disfunctions, you experience body aches and pains, muscle pain, fatigue, inability to heal, brain fog, headaches, and other neurological symptoms such as mood swings.

The Institute for Restorative Health indicates that there are four main points to be mindful of in a mitochondria-healing diet: [8]
1. Healthy fats such as avocados, butter, olive oil, nuts and seeds, coconut oil, fish
2. Phytonutrients – regular consumption of every colour of fruit and vegetable, preferably daily
3. Anti-inflammatory foods – herbs, spices, minimally processed, organic
4. Reduced carbs (no or low grain), and high fiber foods.

It is interesting that that these dietary recommendations also speak to healing the gut.

Heal you gut and get rid of mitochondrial disfunction, which will lead to a good mood and plenty of energy!

Leaky gut not only leads to autoimmune disease, but also contributes to mood disorders, weight gain, skin issues, hormone imbalances and last but not least, brain degeneration.[9]

Let's look at each one of these.

Sources of References in Section 4

1.   https://www.ncbi.nlm.nih.gov/pubmedhealth/PMH0072548/
2.   https://epidemicanswers.org/reference-library/the-immune-system/immune-system-101/
3.   Dr Moodley, Compounding Pharmacy
4.   https://autoimmunewellness.com/what-is-the-role-of-th1-and-th2-in-autoimmune-disease/
5.   https://www.ncbi.nlm.nih.gov/pubmedhealth/PMH0072548/
6.   https://paulaowens.com/heal-autoimmune-disease/
7.   https://www.ncbi.nlm.nih.gov/pmc/articles/PMC5437217/
8.   https://instituteforrestorativehealth.com/2019/06/14/how-to-boost-your-energy-and-restore-your-energy/
9.   http://realfoodcon.com/dr-tom-obryan/

Section 5
Mood Disorders

MOODY AND NOT KNOWING WHY?

I don't know myself – why all these emotions?

In the *Naturopathic Doctor News and Review* it is reported that evidence shows that bowel disorders are often correlated with poor mood. It is alarming that 20% of patients with functional bowel disorders such as irritable bowel syndrome (IBS) have diagnosable psychiatric illness. Even more alarming, almost one-third of patients with Irritable Bowel Syndrome (IBS) have been found to have anxiety or depression.[1]

> Andrew Gaeddert, RH, registered herbalist and the president and founder of Health Concerns, recommends peppermint tea or chamomile tea for treatment of IBS. He also indicates that food allergies, in particular wheat and milk allergies can cause IBS. He recommends removing wheat and dairy from the diet if you have IBS symptoms.

Neurological manifestations such as anxiety or depression in patients with established celiac disease have been reported since 1966. When people with celiac disease eat gluten (a protein found in wheat, rye and barley), their body mounts an immune response that attacks the small intestine. These attacks lead to damage of the stomach lining that leads to nutrient mal absorption. **Damage to the intestinal wall can eventually lead to malnourishment, as well as loss of bone density, miscarriages, infertility and even neurological diseases or even some cancers.**

It was not until 30 years after 1966 that gluten sensitivity was first shown to manifest solely as neurological dysfunction, such as unexplained neuropathies and ataxia. Neuropathy is a disease or dysfunction of one or more peripheral nerves, typically causing numbness or weakness and ataxia is the loss of full control of bodily movements. This is scary don't you think! Gluten sensitivity can cause neuropathy and ataxia!

Celiac is an antibody-mediated disease affecting 1% of the population and is generally characterized by gastrointestinal complaints. **Gluten sensitivities or intolerance can be subtler in reaction, often without overt gastrointestinal problems, manifesting instead as extra-intestinal neurologic and psychiatric symptoms.**

Gluten sensitivity may be even more causative of psychiatric illness than overt celiac disease. According to this review, one study showed gluten withdrawal to produce a greater improvement in gut symptoms in non-celiac, gluten-sensitive patients than in patients with celiac disease (75% vs 64.7%, respectively). [1]

If you have IBS symptoms or any neurological symptoms such as depression, anxiety or even neuropathy, it is worth it to omit gluten and dairy from your diet for three weeks and see what happens! What do you have to lose?

Any food to which a person is sensitive can spark an immune-related response in the digestive tract, eliciting inflammatory cascades throughout the body. This is a very important statement. Take a moment to ponder on it. Any food you are sensitive to can spark an immune related response.

This means it is critical to identify your specific food sensitivities or intolerances.

Stressors will also increase the likelihood of immune response to food by decreasing parasympathetic response and proper enzymatic production. Low digestive enzyme status leads to an inability to digest food, which can then result in undigested macromolecules breaching the intestinal barrier. This, in turn, can cause inflammation in your whole body. Particles that escape from the digestive tract can travel to other parts of the body and trigger global inflammatory effects,

     Your Greatest Wealth is your Health   55

contributing to disease. **If someone has a predisposition (genetically or epigenetically) to a particular disease, leaky gut and its accompanying inflammation may increase the likelihood that this disease will manifest.** For example, in an individual prone to heart problems, inflammation in the coronary arteries will contribute to endothelial dysfunction and blockage. In a person predisposed to autoimmune conditions like rheumatoid arthritis, the inflammation may contribute to disfigured and painful joints.[2]

What this means in plain English, is that eating a food that you are sensitive to, will cause inflammation in your body. This in turn will cause damage to your intestinal wall, which will in turn lead to food particles and impurities entering your blood stream. This in turn can cause large scale inflammation. And subsequently a wide spectrum of illness.

In other words, depending on the weak link in your chain, the cumulative effect of inflammation and leaky gut will affect that area of your body. It differs for all of us as mentioned above. Can you now start to appreciate just how important it is to treat leaky gut? **The good news is that if you avoid such trigger foods, epigenetics kick in, which means you can turn off that "bad" gene and prevent it from manifesting.**

By treating leaky gut, multiple illnesses can be treated by addressing the root cause.

In the Naturopathic Doctor News and Review, it is highlighted that in a similar fashion, people with mood disorders may have a greater tendency to have brain inflammation. When leaky gut and intestinal inflammation are present, intracellularly leaked particles translocate into the bloodstream where they enter the hepatic portal system and spur upregulation of the hepatic Kupffer cells, thereby triggering microglial inflammation in the brain; this can result in brain degeneration and changes in mood.[3]

Perivascular areas of the brain, such as the hypothalamus and limbic system, are especially vulnerable to inflammation and contribute to "sickness behaviour" (anhedonia: the inability to feel pleasure in normally pleasurable activities, fatigue, etc). The likelihood of this cascade of events has been shown to be far greater with leaky gut than when the intestinal barrier is intact.

There are various ways the body reveals increased levels of inflammation. These may include the presence of skin conditions (rashes, eczema, psoriasis, rosacea, etc) or be more internal (such as autoimmune conditions, cancers, cardiovascular disease, mental health, and inflammatory bowel diseases).[4]

Dr Tom O'Bryan makes us aware that a whole new science was developed in 2007 called **enteric neuroscience, which studies how the environment of the gut affects the nerves in the brain.** Now there are hundreds of studies that document that the bacteria in the gut control the production of your nerve hormones (neurotransmitters). **Depression, anxiety, schizophrenia, and any psychoses are being directly associated with an imbalance in the gut bacteria.**

Let's step of mood disorders and focus on stubborn fat.

Sources of References in Section 5

1. https://plantmedicinesummit.com/program/42
2. https://plantmedicinesummit.com/program/42
3. https://plantmedicinesummit.com/program/42
4. http://ndnr.com/anxietydepressionmental-health/mood-and-leaky-gut/

Section 6

Stubborn fat and heart disease

JUST CAN'T GET RID OF THE FAT!

No matter what I do, I can't seem to lose the extra weight

Obesity increases your risk for numerous conditions including heart disease, stroke, Type 2 diabetes, high blood pressure, and cancer.

Globally, obesity now kills about the same number of people as tobacco and more than all wars, terrorism, and violence. **Nearly all people who are overweight already have "pre-diabetes" and have significant risks of disease and death.** They just don't know it. When you begin to put on weight, especially belly fat, your biology shifts out of balance, veering into the unstable and unhealthy territory of disease. This in turn makes you fatter. A vicious, deadly cycle ensues unless you take control of your weight.

Dr Mark Hyman explains that when your body senses foreign invaders (as a result of leaky gut), a specific cascade of events is set off in which your **white blood cells and some special chemicals called cytokines mobilize to protect you. This normal type of inflammation is a good thing.** It helps your body protect and heal itself. However, when your immune system shifts out of balance, inflammation can become out of control, causing a chronic, smouldering fire inside your body that contributes to disease and weight gain.[1]

The causes of this type of inflammation are all around you. The sugar you eat, high doses of the wrong oils and fats in your diet, hidden food allergens, lack of exercise, chronic stress, and hidden infections all trigger a raging, unseen inflammation deep in your cells and tissues.

And this inflammation leads to every one of the major chronic diseases of aging including heart disease, cancer, diabetes, dementia, and more. It's also by far the major contributor to obesity.

Dr Hyman says, "being fat is being inflamed — period!"

Dr Moodley says: 'Fat is composed of inflammatory cells. It is also a storage for toxins. The more toxic you are, the more fat will protect your body."[2]

We are getting closer to the answer.

If you don't address inflammation by eliminating hidden food allergens or sensitivities and by eating an anti-inflammatory diet, you will never succeed at effective and permanent weight loss.

Hidden sensitivities and allergies to food you eat every day are making you ill and obese.

When most people think of food allergies, they usually imagine someone eating a peanut and ending up in the emergency room with a swollen tongue, hives, and not being able to breathe. That's what is called an immediate allergy (also known as an IgE hypersensitivity reaction). This is very serious but not common.

Dr Hyman emphasises that there is a different type of reaction to foods that is much less dramatic and deadly but still of great concern. It is called a delayed allergy (or IgG delayed hypersensitivity reaction). This reaction is much more common and creates a lot of suffering for millions of people. It's mostly ignored by conventional medicine, yet it plays a HUGE role in many chronic illnesses and weight problems.

Again, I need you to ponder this issue. We always think we should have an immediate response if we are intolerant to a food. This is not true. It is crucial to monitor your bodily

responses and moods after eating certain foods for at least 3 days after.

This type of delayed allergic reaction can cause symptoms anywhere from a few hours to a few days after ingestion. It also causes a wide range of problems like weight gain, fluid retention, fatigue, brain fog, irritable bowel syndrome, mood problems, headaches, sinus and nasal congestion, joint pains, acne, eczema, and more. Gluten is one of those![3]

Dr Hyman says getting rid of this fluid by reducing inflammation is a good thing. It is what will allow your body to start the healing process so you can achieve permanent weight loss and optimal health.

Consuming a low-allergy diet for just 1 week will help you eliminate the excess swelling and fluid that accumulates in your tissues from food-induced chronic inflammation. It is interesting that Dr Hyman says despite criticisms you may have heard about losing ONLY water weight, this is essential for your body to begin to heal and detoxify. And the side effect is that you lose significant weight quickly and safely.

Dr Hyman indicates that in his practice, treating food allergies and improving nutrition in general is the single most powerful tool he uses to treat, reverse, and even cure hundreds of diseases that conventional medicine fails at miserably.

These include allergies, arthritis, autoimmune diseases, fatigue, sinus problems, hormonal disorders, obesity, high blood pressure, cholesterol, digestive diseases like irritable bowel syndrome, reflux, and colitis, and even mood disorders like depression and anxiety to just to name a few.

Dr Hyman makes a profound statement: We are seeing an epidemic of inflammatory diseases. In fact, nearly every modern disease, everything from autoimmune diseases, heart disease, and cancer to obesity, diabetes, and dementia is caused by inflammation!

He emphasises that while everyone is different, there are some foods that irritate the immune system more than others. They are gluten (wheat, barley, rye, oats, spelt, kamut), dairy (milk, cheese, butter, yogurt), corn, eggs, soy, nuts, nightshades (tomatoes, bell peppers, potatoes, eggplant), citrus, and yeast (baker's yeast, brewer's yeast, and fermented products).

Please stop for a moment and think about these. Your first step would be to become more aware of how these foods are perhaps affecting you. This is your first step to healing.

For more than 50 percent of us, there are some foods that just don't agree with us and prevent vibrant, good health.

The easiest and most cost-effective way to confirm if you have food allergies is to follow an elimination diet.

This means you get rid of the top "trouble" foods as listed above for 2 to 4 weeks, then reintroduce them one at a time and see what happens. Eliminating foods that cause allergic reactions or sensitivities is the basis for the remarkable results people have, like losing weight, feeling better, and getting rid of chronic symptoms. The top foods to start with are gluten, dairy and sugar.

The Compounding Pharmacy of South Africa published some guidelines for an elimination diet...these can be downloaded here:
https://www.compounding.co.za/wp-content/uploads/2017/02/Comprehensive-Elimination-Diet.pdf

In as little as a week or less people notice dramatic relief from all the symptoms.

Dr Hyman says that simply put, your diet, the way you live, and the medications you take are to blame.

They all injure your gut. **They change the bacteria and damage the gut's lining, which is the critical barrier that keeps your immune system from having to deal with all the garbage, toxins, and allergens inside your intestinal tract. This damage is called a leaky gut.** Food particles "leak" across the damaged barrier and your immune system (60 percent of which is right under that lining) starts to attack these partially digested food particles. That's when you develop food intolerances or allergies.[4]

Just because you have a food allergy or intolerance doesn't mean you have to suffer with it. In fact, there's a lot you can do to deal with the problem, rebalance your system, and eliminate chronic symptoms. You can take charge of your health!

Can you believe it is this simple? Well, I am living proof! It is that simple. My biggest trouble food has been gluten. I thought I could get away with having less gluten. That is unfortunately not true. I urge you to give it a try. Remove ALL gluten from your diet for 3 weeks and see how you feel. But be sure to check your food labels for hidden gluten especially in spices, meats, sauces and soup mixes. More guidance will be provided later in this book.

Dr Mark Hyman also goes into more detail on belly fat. He indicates that Insulin is the key player in belly fat.

Numerous hormones contribute to belly fat, but none proves more powerful than insulin, your fat storage hormone. Too high levels of insulin (because of overindulgence), cause your body to gain weight around the belly, and you become more apple-shaped over time. High insulin levels also drive inflammation and oxidative stress, creating myriad of other symptoms.

Eventually you become insulin resistant, which leads your body to generate even more belly fat, but now it becomes stubborn fat. Fatigue after meals, sugar cravings, blood sugar swings or hypoglycaemia, high triglycerides, low HDL and low sex drive. Problems with blood clotting are also common among people who are overweight.

Less insulin equals less belly fat, since too much insulin makes you hungry and stores belly fat. The best thing you can do is to lose weight. It's important to note that high insulin levels don't just exist in a vacuum. They influence other hormones like leptin which is your satiety (hunger) hormone. When insulin blocks leptin, your body thinks it is starving even after a burger, fries, and a soda. Ever wonder how you can still be hungry right after a big meal? It is the insulin surge and the leptin resistance.

More than any other food, sugar becomes responsible for hijacking your brain chemistry and your metabolism to create insulin resistance and all its repercussions. Sugar is different from other calories that come from protein, fat, or non-starchy carbs such as greens.

Sugar scrambles all your normal appetite controls. The more sugar you eat, the more sugar you want to eat. And the more belly fat you accumulate.

I am sure you wondering, but what about fructose?

Dr Hyman says fructose is the most metabolically damaging form of sugar. It goes right to your liver, where it starts manufacturing fat, which triggers more insulin resistance and causes chronically elevated blood insulin levels, driving your body to store everything you eat as fat. And guess what, it stores around your belly. You also get a fatty liver, which generates more inflammation. Chronic inflammation causes more weight gain. Anything that causes inflammation will worsen insulin resistance. See this vicious cycle?[5]

Another problem with fructose is that it doesn't send informational feedback to the brain, signalling that a load of calories just hit the body. Nor does it reduce ghrelin, the appetite hormone that is usually reduced when you eat real food. We are programmed to store belly fat in response to sugar so that we can survive the winter when food is scarce. Genes do play a role, but they are a minor contributor to the massive obesity and diabetes pandemic we are facing globally. By shutting down the insulin surges, you can combat belly fat storage and cravings.[6]

Below are a few tips provided by Dr Hyman. In this programme you will receive a comprehensive plan that can transform your health.

1. **Eat real (whole) food.** When we eat real foods / whole foods, which contain many nutrients, we are more satisfied, eat less, and lose belly fat. Getting adequate vitamins and minerals helps you burn calories more efficiently, helps regulate appetite, lowers inflammation, boosts detoxification, aids digestion, regulates stress hormones, and helps your cells become more insulin sensitive. Along with lots of green vegetables, include protein in every meal since studies show it keeps you fuller longer so you lose more weight.

2. **Manage stress levels.** Chronic stress causes your brain to shrink and your belly to grow. Dr Hyman says that in treating patients with insulin resistance or diabetes they always see chronically elevated levels of the stress hormone cortisol causing increased blood sugar and cholesterol, depression, dementia, and promotes the accumulation of stubborn fat. They crave sugar and carbs and seek comfort food.

3. **Address food sensitivities**. What I found very interesting is that he says that we often crave the very foods we are allergic to. Getting off them is not easy, but after two to three days without them, you will have renewed energy, relief from cravings and symptoms, and begin to shed belly fat. Gluten and dairy are two big food sensitivities, but many others can create roadblocks that make losing belly fat nearly impossible.

4. **Get enough sleep.** Not getting enough sleep drives sugar and carb cravings by affecting your appetite hormones. One study found even a partial night's poor sleep could contribute to insulin resistance. Poor sleep also adversely impacts fat-regulating hormones like leptin and ghrelin.

5. **Optimize your nutrient levels:** Take a high-quality multivitamin that contains blood sugar-balancing nutrients.

6. **Optimize omega-3 fat.** Omega-3 fatty acids are important for controlling insulin function.

7. **Optimize your vitamin D levels** as this critical vitamin supports appetite control.

8. **Consider taking natural supplements for cravings control.** L-glutamine and PGX (a super fiber) are among the natural dietary supplements that can help reduce cravings.

9. **Monitor alcohol.** Drinking alcohol as a daily habit, alcohol can do more harm than you realize, especially if you have diabetes or struggle with weight loss. Consider this: If you drink two glasses of wine a day, you will consume about 72,000 extra calories a year, which could mean an extra 20 pounds a year. And these liquid calories go straight to your belly. Stop for six weeks. See how you feel. Then, if you want, enjoy one to three glasses of wine or alcohol a week.

10. **Exercise regularly:** Aside from changing your diet, exercise is probably the single best medication for obesity. Walk at least 30 minutes every day.

Now that we looked at weight gain, let's move to brain degeneration.

Sources of References in Section 6

1. http://drhyman.com/blog/2012/01/27/inflammation-how-to-cool-the-fire-inside-you-thats-making-you-fat-and-diseased/
2. Dr Moodley, Compounding Pharmacy, Bryanston
3. http://drhyman.com/blog/2012/01/27/inflammation-how-to-cool-the-fire-inside-you-thats-making-you-fat-and-diseased/
4. http://drhyman.com/blog/2012/01/27/inflammation-how-to-cool-the-fire-inside-you-thats-making-you-fat-and-diseased/
5. http://drhyman.com/blog/2012/01/27/inflammation-how-to-cool-the-fire-inside-you-thats-making-you-fat-and-diseased/
6. http://drhyman.com/blog/2015/01/29/7-ways-permanently-banish-belly-fat/

Section 7
Brain Degeneration

I AM GETTING OLD; I CANNOT REMEMBER AS WELL AS I USED TO

Becoming forgetful as your grow older is NOT normal!

You will be surprised just how significant the impact of your diet is on your brain health. When your gut wall is in bad shape, it is not only your body that gets inflamed, your brain also gets inflamed.

Dr Mark Hyman has published his Broken Brain series in January 2018.[1] As mentioned before, in this series he unpacks the link between the gut and the brain. He looks at food allergies, stress, medical drugs and environmental toxins, and the impact thereof on the gut. Dr Hyman treats patients with multiple brain issues such as Dementia, MS, Alzheimer's, Fibromyalgia, Schizophrenia, Anxiety and Depression through addressing their gut health. He talks about Schizophrenia patients that are following a normal lifestyle after diet changes. Living a normal life, without medication, released from an institution. Yes, believe it!

It must be noted that you should not stop taking prescribed medication without consulting your doctor, functional health practitioner, homeopath or an integrative health practitioner

He highlights that medical drugs such as anti-inflammatory, non-steroidal drugs and acid blockers can damage the gut. As well as environmental toxicity and stress.

Later in this book, environmental toxicity and healthy alternatives will be dealt with in great detail, as well as stress management and impact of medicines on the gut.

His Broken Brain Series will revolutionise the way we look at brain degeneration. I would highly recommend you acquire and listen to this series when he addresses the gut brain connection.

He refers a new wave of research around Psycho-neuro-immune-endocrinology. It refers to the link between one's thoughts, your nervous system, immune system and endocrine system. No part of the body stands alone. Every single part interacts with the rest. The problem starts when the immune or nervous systems overreact to normal substances like food particles.

He highlights that 3 reactions to foods trigger brain injury, namely:

1. Inflammation in the body which in turn creates inflammation in the brain
2. Peptides (from wheat gluten and casein protein in dairy) disturb neurotransmitters. Neurotransmitters are often referred to as the body's chemical messengers
3. Excitotoxins that increases glutamate (MSG), overexcite the brain and ultimately kill brain cells

Processed foods remain loaded with excitotoxins, all of which have been linked to brain cell death, infertility, problems with sexual development, violent behaviours, and hormonal disorders.

He emphasises that an unhappy forgetful brain is an inflamed brain.

He says that what inflames the brain, inflames the gut and what inflames the gut inflames the brain.

Thus, addressing inflammation in the gut, directly addresses inflammation in the brain.

Great emphasis is put on the inflammatory effects of gluten. He highlights that Dr Fasano has done extensive research on gluten sensitivity and indicates that **everyone's gut gets damaged from eating gluten.**[2]

In this series, he and a host of experts recommend that everyone removes gluten from their diet.

It is emphasised that an anti-inflammatory diet should be followed, and a great variety of foods should be consumed. Eating the same foods every day should be avoided. He also highlights the importance of proper detoxification of the body. His key message is "what you do to the body affects the brain, and what you do to the brain, affects the body!"

In the Broken Brain docuseries, Dr. David Musnick says one of the best ways to heal head injuries is to lower inflammation in the diet. To do that, he says, you "decrease fried foods, breaded foods, and eliminate all trans fats in the diet."

Later in this book, we will address the impact of your thoughts on your body.

For now, please appreciate that your brain health can be significantly improved through a healthy diet, reducing environmental toxins, exercise, and reducing stress.

Dr Hyman says that crucial supplements for brain health are:

- Multivitamin / Mineral
- Magnesium
- Vitamin D3 (2000 IU a day and maybe more if you're deficient - check with your healthcare practitioner)
- Methylated B complex vitamins
- Omega-3 fats (EPA & DHA from fish oil)

Let's move to the impact of leaky gut on the skin.

Sources of References in Section 7

1. https://brokenbrain.com/02-gut-brain/
2. https://brokenbrain.com/

Section 8

Skin Disorders, Allergies and MCS

NO MATTER WHAT I DO, MY SKIN IS A MESS!

I've tried everything!

Dr Trevor Cates, in the Healthy Gut Experts Summit (Jan 2018), emphasizes the link between the gut and skin disorders. Dr. Trevor Cates is author of the bestselling book Clean Skin From Within. She believes in inner and outer nourishment, avoiding toxic ingredients.

In other words, whatever you feed yourself with or put on your skin, should be natural and non-toxic.[1]

Skin disorders, especially on your face, have a detrimental effect on self-esteem. It is crucial to realise that a skin disorder is a symptom of something else. It is a sign that something is wrong in your body. It typically traces back to leaky gut.

Sources of poor skin include:

- Nutritional deficiencies, which is a result of leaky gut
- Gut microbiome in-balance. There is a direct link between the gut and your skin.

She indicates that by treating the gut microbiome, many skin issues are resolved. But one cannot ignore external factors such as personal care products being used on the outside of the skin.

> Her approach is summarised as:
>
> 1. **Clean plate** – eating food that would nourish you and that are anti-inflammatory and organic. Avoiding trigger foods that leads to inflammation.
> 2. **Clean slate** – This has to do with the products we use directly on our bodies that could impact our health due to their toxic nature. It has to be free of hormone disrupting chemicals.
> 3. **Clean body** – This element looks at other environmental toxins such as air quality, fumes from cleaning chemicals etc that could impact your health.
> 4. **Clean mind** – The last item refers to stress and the ability to manage stress effectively. Stress is a reality and enhances performance. But excessive, chronic stress can be very harmful.

She emphasises the importance of developing healthy habits that would transform your health for the rest of your life.[2]

Key trigger foods for skin issues

She highlights that **sugar** or any foods that turn into sugar, and increase blood sugar, can lead to glycation issues. Glucose binds with proteins in the body. In the case of skin, we talk about collagen. Collagen helps with skin elasticity. When glycation happens, our collagen becomes more rigid and less elastic which leads to wrinkles and sagging skin. Sugar also increases insulin. Insulin spikes can trigger excess androgen activity which could lead to acne breakouts. Hence the importance to balance blood sugar.

> **Collagen** - We all need collagen for good health. Collagen rich foods or supplements can be very helpful in healing gut permeability, as well as supporting skin and joints.

Dr Karen Lee indicates that food allergies have a major impact on eczema. She says that eczema is common in children and symptoms are likely to manifest on the elbows, knees, neck folds, behind the eyes and above the eye lids, and above the buttocks.[3]

She highlights that the body can heal itself if we support it by removing bad triggers such as processed sugar.

- **Natural sugar** such as maple syrup and honey is best. She highlights that cancer thrives on sugar.

- **Eliminate all processed food** or anything synthetically made such as artificial colours and flavours.

- **Repairing the gut lining** is crucial, such as bone broth and using a good quality probiotic or eating foods rich in pre- and probiotics.

- She says that if you **eat resistant starches** such as potato, it is best to cook it and let it cool. It reduces the starch level.

- **Fermented foods** are also highly recommended.

- As well as **drinking filtered room temperature water** first thing in the morning. Stay hydrated.

Another culprit is gluten. If you battle with skin issues, remove gluten from your diet for two weeks and see if you experience an improvement

What about allergies?

When the sneezing, sniffling, and runny eyes of springtime kick in, most people grab for the allergy pills, antihistamines, and eye drops. But did you know you can greatly relieve if not banish your allergy symptoms by fixing your gut?

It may sound crazy that your gut health would affect your sinuses, but in fact the two systems are very intertwined. *Both the respiratory tract and the digestive tract are immune barriers, meaning it's their job to protect the body from outside invaders.*

The gut, in particular, profoundly influences the entire immune system. When gut health suffers, so does the rest of your body, and the result for many people are allergy symptoms that flare up each spring.

If you want soft, young-looking skin, she recommends making these tips the core of your beauty ritual. Interestingly enough, it will also greatly support the reduction of allergy symptoms.

1. **Bone Broth**

   Wrinkles form when your skin breaks down. To erase these wrinkles, you need to boost your collagen levels. Bone broth is the most collagen-rich food source on the planet, so drink up! It's far more effective than even the most expensive wrinkle creams. The recipe will follow later in the book

2. **Omega-3-rich foods**

   Think of aging skin cells as slightly deflated balls. Omega-3 fatty acids fill up the walls of these cells, making them bouncy again. To get plenty of omega-3's, eat fatty fish and walnuts or take a high-quality omega-3 supplement.

3. **Amino acids**

   Amino acids are the building blocks of collagen and elastin, which are vital to healthy skin. A diet high in essential amino acids (which the body can't make on its own) keeps your skin firm and "elastic" while a deficiency makes it thin and dry. Meat and eggs are your best sources for essential amino acids.

4. **Potassium-rich foods**

   She suggests switching from regular table salt to sea salt. Regular salt pulls water out of your cells, leaving them "flabby" and promoting wrinkles. But sea salt, which is high in potassium, does just the opposite: It pulls water into your cells, making them firm. You can also get skin-hydrating potassium from fruits and veggies, nuts, meat, poultry, and fish. Himalayan salt is also a great alternative.

---

5. Fermented foods

A healthy gut translates into radiant and wrinkle-free skin, while a sick gut is a leading cause of skin aging. That's because good gut bacteria help keep your body well supplied with the nutrients your skin thrives on. Bad bacteria, on the other hand, can cause leaky gut syndrome, allowing toxins to escape your intestines and create inflammation throughout your body. As a result, your skin looks old. To improve your gut health, eat fermented foods like kefir and sauerkraut.

6. Green and yellow vegetables

Vegetables are loaded with skin-protecting antioxidants, which help prevent oxidative stress (damage to cells caused by free radicals). A higher intake of green and yellow vegetables (along with a higher intake of healthy fats) reduces wrinkling.

7. Green tea

Green tea is also loaded with antioxidants. Research shows that it protects your skin against sun damage, which is the primary cause of wrinkles.

8. Phytoceramides

Ceramides are a naturally occurring constituent of skin that keeps it hydrated. Phytoceramides, found in beets and spinach, offer similar benefits.

What about multiple chemical sensitivities?[4]

Multiple chemical sensitivity (MCS), sometimes called environmental illness, is becoming much more common. In fact, it affects millions today, though some of these people are totally unaware they are affected. *MCS is characterized by allergic reactions to a wide range of foods, chemical odours, even electrical fields and other phenomena.*[5] Chemical sensitivity often develops after an exposure to a toxic substance, or after an infection or other illness. Symptoms may include virtually anything. Chemical sensitivity can mimic other illnesses and can contribute to the development of other disorders.

I had severe chemical sensitivities ... I literally reacted to everything! With MCS one also has an acute sense of smell. Someone would walk past me and I would smell the washing detergent on their clothes, or their deodorant. Or I would walk into a restaurant and need to walk out as the chemicals used to clean the floor were just too strong for me to cope with. I would experience extreme discomfort, itching, little sores would appear on my head and in my neck immediately after any exposure, my eyes would swell and become very dry. It always felt like I had sand in my eyes.

Once I treated my gut with the protocols explained in this book, my sensitivities went away. Today I may get a severe exposure to, for instance, pesticides, and I feel very ill for an hour or two, but with certain interventions, the symptoms disappear very quickly. If you have chemical sensitivities, I want to encourage you not to give up! There is hope! I suffered with severe chemical sensitivities. For a very long time I did not know that I had chemical sensitivities. Once I knew what it was, I was able to take action. The three main factors that improve chemical sensitivities are:

1. Eating a clean, whole food diet
2. Healing your gut and keeping it healthy
3. Removing environmental toxins (refer to section 17 for a lot of detail!)

I hope that by now you can start to appreciate just how important your gut health is. It is at the root of almost all diseases.

It may blow your mind that treating leaky gut can improve, if not arrest, so many diseases.

But what about hormone imbalances?

Sources of References in Section 8

1. https://healthygutexperts.com/day-1/drtrevor/
2. https://healthygutexperts.com/day-1/drtrevor/
3. https://healthygutexperts.com/day-4/karen-lee/
4. https://healthygutexperts.com/day-4/karen-lee/
5. https://www.drkellyann.com/science-collagen-supplementation/

Section 9

Hormone imbalances

MY HORMONES ARE ALL OVER THE SHOW!

I am sick of taking pills for my hormones and it just makes me feel worse!

Wellness and vitality expert, Dr Shelena C. Lalji, M.D. ("Dr Shel"), helps her patients regain their healthy balance so they can look and feel their best.

She highlights that women in their thirties and forties, go into oestrogen dominance which can lead to a host of symptoms such as hair loss, insomnia, weight gain and so forth.

She says that in treating patients with hormone issues, she always starts with the gut.

> Some aspects she addresses in her treatment include:[1]
> 1. Healthy eating
> 2. Enough sleep
> 3. Keeping hydrated - drinking water
> 4. Stress management

Dr Anna Cabeca indicates that women regularly suffer with vaginal dryness, pain and yeast infections. She references a patient that suffered from chronic vaginal irritation. No bacterial infections could be found. They then changed her diet to gluten free and dairy free, and her symptoms radically improved.[2]

Dr Amy Day says there are interrelations between the gut function and hormone function.

> She indicates that healing the gut (microbiome) has a direct impact on improvement of vaginal health. Intermittent fasting is crucial for gut health. As well as spending time in nature.

Dr Osborne highlights that grains disrupt hormone balances. He highlights that sleep disturbances, hot flushes, headaches, poor libido, hair loss and fatigue can all be as a result of gluten intolerance.[3]

Dr Osborne furthermore highlights the five hormones impacted by grains and what the impacts are:

1. **Thyroid disruption** causes weight gain, muscle pain, and emotional pain when we start losing our hair, libido, and daily motivation.
2. **Adrenal hormone** disruption leads to pain by increasing inflammation, blood sugar levels, causing water retention, weight gain, and severe fatigue.
3. **Insulin hormone** disruption causes blood sugar problems, lowering energy and increasing our risk of developing Diabetes and Dementia.
4. **Estrogen and Progesterone** disruption contributes to the pain of increased menstrual cramping, breast tenderness, increased risk of cancers, and infertility.
5. **Testosterone disruption** can contribute to weight gain, severe fatigue, memory problems, as well as loss of muscle and motivation.

I am sure that the different puzzle pieces are starting to form a very clear picture in your mind. Our gut health is at the core of our overall health.

By addressing symptoms, we may just take one pill that causes another health issue. But by addressing gut health, many of these illnesses can be prevented or successfully treated.

At this point I want you to stop and listen carefully!

By now you may feel a bit overwhelmed. Being faced with these realities could potentially cause you to feel either paralysed or obsessed.

Those of you that feel paralysed want to ignore these facts and pretend they do not exist. You do not know where to start. Those of you that feel obsessed, want to go overboard and only eat or drink certain foods, perhaps lock yourself in your home and prevent any environmental exposure. Do not ignore these emotions. But note that neither of these responses are going to be good for you.

There is a solution. Once you have raised your self-awareness on how foods and toxins affect you, you can take charge of your own health.

You can make better choices that directly affect your health for the better.

What I need to emphasize now and will do again later in this book, is that you must take control of what is within your power. You can't control everything.

But there are things you can control. You can also not change everything at once. It will be overwhelming. Making one change at a time and seeing the impact of such a change is the best way to go about it. Especially once we start making food and drink choices, please do not stop eating all food and only eat one or two types of healthy foods. **Remember, too much of a good thing is always bad for you!** When it comes to food choices, moderation and variety is key!!! This book will guide you step by step...Do not make too many changes at one time, tackle it at the pace that works for you.

We will come back to these principles later in the book. Now, let's start your journey.

Sources of References in Section 9

1. https://healthygutexperts.com/day-2/dr-shel-lalji/
2. https://healthygutexperts.com/day-5/dr-anna-cabeca/
3. https://www.glutenfreesociety.org/the-gluten-hydra-hormones-the-medical-trap/

     Your Greatest Wealth is your Health   81

Section 10
Functional Medicine

THE SOLUTION

My health is my greatest wealth

As a solution, I would like to introduce you to the Functional Medicine Model.

The Functional Medicine Model is an individualized, patient-centered, science-based approach that empowers patients and practitioners to work together to address the underlying causes of disease and promote optimal wellness. It requires a detailed understanding of each person's genetic, biochemical, and lifestyle factors and leverages that data to direct personalised treatment plans that lead to improved patient outcomes.

By addressing root cause, rather than symptoms, practitioners can successfully treat and prevent disease. They may find one condition has many different causes and, likewise, one cause may result in many different conditions.[1]

According to the Functional Medicine Institute, a properly functioning digestive system is critical to good health. In fact, problems with the gastrointestinal (GI) tract can cause more than just stomach aches or diarrhoea. As we have seen, GI issues may lead to several other chronic health problems that seem unrelated to digestive health, including autoimmune diseases such as rheumatoid arthritis and type 1 diabetes, skin problems such as eczema and acne, rosacea, depression, and heart disease (just to name a few).

The functional medicine approach addresses the 5Rs, namely: remove, replace, reinoculate, repair, and rebalance.

When applied to various chronic problems, the 5R-programme can lead to dramatic improvement in symptoms, and sometimes even complete resolution of the problem. I know you may feel quite frustrated and disheartened right now. You may feel that the whole world has failed you and that you can't see the light at the end of the tunnel.

Guess what, I have news for you!! You can and will feel much better! Once you know the root cause of your illness, you can arrest your symptoms. Up to this point you have already raised your self-awareness by at least 100%. This knowledge will empower you to make the changes you need.

At this point I must emphasize, a lot of what you will be exposed to in this 5R programme, you may at first think is nonsense. Trust me, it is not. It has all been researched and I have tried and tested every one of these strategies. I am living proof. It is now time to open your mind to new ideas. Be willing to try these strategies. You have nothing to lose. Only a LOT to gain! You will not believe what impact dietary changes and lifestyle changes can have on your overall health! And before we get into the nuts and bolts of the programme, also know that the more of these you apply in your life, the quicker your progress will be. A holistic approach to reducing one's toxic load renders amazing results. That said, to avoid being overwhelmed, it is best to approach it in a step-by-step manner. If you remove the big triggers, you will feel like a different person.

**Keep your mind open and keep up your commitment
to be a better, healthier you! You can do it!!!**

The elements of the 5R-programme are described briefly below.

1. **Remove** stressors: get rid of things that negatively affect the environment of the gastro-intestinal tract including allergic foods and parasites or other bad bugs such as bacteria or yeast. This might involve using an allergy "elimination diet" to find out what foods are causing symptoms or it may involve taking drugs or herbs to eradicate a particular bug. It also means removing toxins from your environment, as well as emotional sterssors.

2. **Replace** digestive secretions: add back things like digestive enzymes, hydrochloric acid, and bile acids that are required for proper digestion and that may be compromised by diet, drugs, diseases, aging, or other factors. Digestive enzymes support healthy digestion and helps break down nutrients you ingest. Hydrochloric acid is naturally created in your stomach. It is the main thing that creates the acidic environment to break down food. If you're deficient in hydrochloric acid, and stomach acid itself, that's not going to allow you to fully digest and break down things like protein, which over time can also cause leaky gut. Reduced bile acid levels in the gut is associated with bacteria overgrowth and inflammation.

   Replace also refers ot replacing all the bad emotions as well as environmnetal toxins with throughst and products that are good for you, which will in turn have a psoitive effect on your gut and health.

3. **Reinoculate** - Help beneficial bacteria flourish by ingesting probiotic foods or supplements that contain the so- called "good" GI bacteria such as bifidobacteria and lactobacillus species, and by consuming the high soluble fiber foods that good bugs like to eat, called "prebiotics." Probiotics are beneficial micro-organisms found in the gut that are also called "friendly bacteria." Use of antibiotics kills both good and bad bacteria. Probiotics in the form of supplements or food are needed to re-inoculate the gut. Fermented foods, such as plain yogurt, sauerkraut, and kombucha are food sources of probiotics. Prebiotics are non-digestible food ingredients that selectively stimulate the growth of beneficial microorganisms already in the colon. In other words, prebiotics feed probiotics. Prebiotics are available in many foods that contain a fiber called inulin, including artichokes, garlic, leeks, onion, chicory, tofu, and other soy products.

    Your Greatest Wealth is your Health   84

4. **Repair** – Help the lining of the gastro-intestinal (GI) tract repair itself by supplying key nutrients that can often be in short supply in a disease state, such as zinc, antioxidants (e.g. vitamins A, C, and E), fish oil, and the amino acid glutamine. We ultimately want to support your microbiome to be in perfect shape at all times.

5. **Rebalance** – Pay attention to lifestyle choices – sleep, exercise and stress can all affect the GI tract.

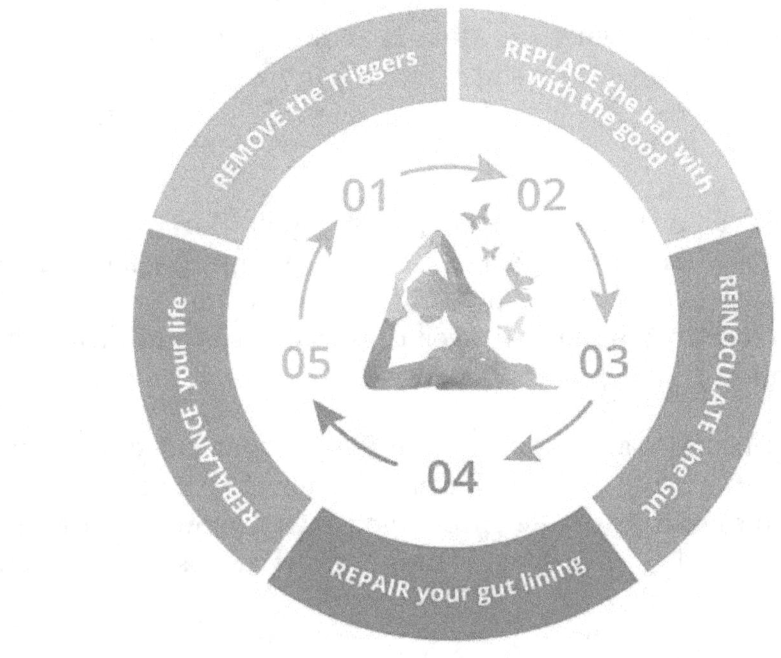

Before we unpack the 5Rs, you need to understand the dynamics of habits.

Sources of References in Section 10

1. https://www.ifm.org/functional-medicine/

     Your Greatest Wealth is your Health

Section 11
Lifestyle Changes

HABITS, YOUR WORST ENEMY OR BEST FRIEND?

Lifestyle changes require habit changes

We all have our weaknesses. Mine is comfort food. Some people escape using alcohol, others smoke, some eat their frustrations away and some use drugs. Reality is that all of these could cumulatively kill you over time.

Let's take alcohol abuse. Alcohol depletes vitamin B from your body and changes your body's metabolism, for some people more than others. Using alcohol can be addictive. Through continuous use, it eventually destroys brain and liver cells which cause difficulty in concentration.

Smoking (nicotine) affects the oxygen flow in your blood and thus negatively affects body cells. It depletes vitamin C from your body. It also dulls the brain. And ladies, in case you did not know, it does cause wrinkles. Smoking is a major cause of heart disease, cancer, emphysema and colds.

Given our incredibly rushed lifestyles, we need to cope at all times. As a result, we tend to turn to painkillers more often than is good for us. The overuse of Paracetamol-based painkillers is toxic to the liver. Painkillers can cause digestive problems, and ironically, it can cause headaches!

I don't like using this example, because it is one of my weaknesses, but too much coffee is not good for you. One or two cups a day is fine for some of us. You need to know that especially when you are stressed, you need to avoid adrenalin stimulants such as coffee and chocolate. They wreak havoc with your blood glucose levels, aggravate heartburn and will make your irritable bowel worse. Caffeine is also a diuretic. That is why you are often warned that drinking too much coffee leads to dehydration.

All these bad habits put strain on your body, which impacts your ability to deal with stress. A healthy body is much more able to cope with constant stress and pressure, than one that is loaded with toxins.

Whatever you use to escape, just know that habits can become addictions, and addictions will harm you. You know your poor habits.

> But remember that to change a habit you need to consistently replace your bad habit with a good one for at least 21 consecutive days, after which the new habit will take root.

Know what you are doing to yourself and do something about it!

There are good habits and bad ones. Regardless of what anyone may tell you, it is much easier to develop a bad habit than it is to develop a good habit. One can learn a bad habit over night, but it takes at least three weeks (21 consecutive days) to develop a good habit. If you want to achieve success, keep it up for six weeks. For instance, if you started a new habit such as a daily walk and you skip one day, you need to start again at day one. Otherwise you will run the risk of falling back into your old habits. Good habits are only set in concrete if you practice them religiously for three to six weeks every day. You only need to do this for the first month or so, after that, even if you deviate from your habit, you will feel the instinctive need to go back to it. Because people differ, some establish habits quicker than others. To be on the safe side, keep it up for six weeks.

Many years ago, I vowed to live a healthier life. One of the habits I had to master was drinking six to eight glasses of water every day. At that stage I was lucky if I drank one glass a day. To make it easier on myself, and having studied the dynamics of habits, I started drinking a glass of water with every other drink I had. Every time I drank a cup of coffee, I also drank a glass of water. For every glass of wine I had, I drank a glass of water. I also decided to drink a glass of water with every meal I ate. By linking the water to existing habits that had already been established, I made it much easier for myself. After three meals and three cups of coffee, I already reached my minimum quota of water for the day. I am happy to say that to this day I am addicted to water. As I am sitting here in front of my laptop, I have my bottle of water next to my computer.

> Please realise that you can't lose or drop a habit. Your best chance of getting rid of a bad habit is replacing it with another habit. You can capitalise on old habits by re-introducing new ones.

For example, if you want to stop smoking, you'll need to exchange your smoking habit with another habit, such as sucking on a mint. Or my favourite subject: if you want to quit eating too many chocolates, you need to replace it with something healthy such as nuts (not peanuts) or fruit. If you try to just quit without replacing the bad habit with a good one, chances are you will go back to your bad habit. The process, as with everything else, starts with self-awareness. **You need to know what you want or need to change.** You may not always be keen to let go of your bad habits, but sometimes you do not have a choice, especially when your health suffers as result of your poor habits. To get back to my water drinking example: I soon replaced drinking coffee almost altogether with drinking water instead. You need to find out what works for you! Perhaps you enjoy some fresh ginger in water, or a slice of lemon, or cucumber. Personalise these tips for you and implement what will work for you!

The last bit of advice I would like to leave you with in regards to habits, is to choose your words. For example, instead of telling yourself and everyone else that you want to "give up" smoking, rather say that you would like to "free yourself from this bad habit for your own good". It will also help align your thinking, which will help you persevere in your quest. As for your journey, decide why you want to do this. If someone then asks you why you don't eat gluten, you can say: "I want to thrive, and gluten keeps me from that goal!"

Remember to link new habits to existing behaviour patterns or habits. Routine is very important. Routine removes stress and brings a sense of being in control. Replace bad habits with good ones. And choose your words in changing your habits.

Let me illustrate through one more example. If you always have barbeque on a Friday, why not eat chicken instead of red meat, make sure to have some gluten free snacks available instead of the standard packet of crisps, have your gluten free bread ready for your "braai broodjie" (grilled sandwich). By working with your habits rather than against them, you can make this journey much easier.

Part of your new habits should be aimed at helping you detox. It is crucial to get rid of all the toxin build up in your body.

Too aggressive detox can be very harmful.

The best approach is to develop lifestyle habits that will clear your body naturally on a continuous basis. These changes should become lifestyle changes. It should be kept up for life.

Making these changes will take time. You will not make these changes over night. You need to implement these changes at the pace that is good for you. And do not allow yourself to be overwhelmed. Making one change and seeing the benefit will motivate you to make the next one.

REMEMBER: One step at a time, one day at a time.

In the next sections, we will unpack the 5Rs in more detail.

Section 12
Remove

REMOVE THE TRIGGERS - INFLAMMATORY FOODS AND TOXINS

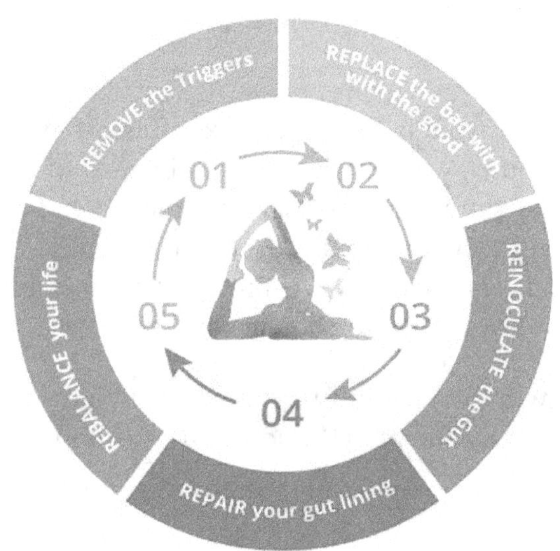

Energy and vitality at your fingertips

Avoid the top inflammatory foods

Every function in our body is controlled by what genes get turned on and off. The key is to turn on genes that leads to health. In other words, foods that are anti-inflammatory. Dr O'Bryan says: "Food selections we make should turn on the anti-inflammatory genes, the heal and repair genes." Stop for a moment and think just how profound this statement is. In Section 13 we will go through inflammatory foods in detail.[1]

Sugar and fruit sugar

Dr Mark Hyman interviewed multiple experts in the Broken Brain docuseries that emphasised that sugar can dramatically alter your metabolism and your brain chemistry, causing you to suffer intense cravings while increasing your risk for disease.[2]

Vicky Konlinger said "Sugar is very pro-inflammatory and one of the things we are learning more and more every day is how much sugar and inflammation are linked to chronic illness, whether it be heart disease or diabetes, but also linked to neurological problems including depression, anxiety, and autism,"

The scary part is that sugar is everywhere.

Try and limit processed foods, desserts and snacks with excess sugar. Also read labels of gluten free products, many of them are loaded with sugar or other flavourings to improve the taste.

Also do not eat excess fruit sugar. Berries, avocados, lemons, peaches, watermelon and nectarines are low in fructose and can be enjoyed, all other fruits should be eaten in moderation. Apples are also considered low in sugar.[3] All fruit juices are highly concentrated and should only be consumed when diluted with water.

Common Cooking Oils

Sunflower, canola, safflower, soy, corn and cottonseed. These oils promote inflammation and are made with cheaper ingredients. Rather use coconut oil or olive oil. We will talk more about this in the next section.

Trans Fats

Trans fats increase bad cholesterol, promote inflammation, obesity and resistance to insulin. They are in fried foods, fast foods, commercially baked goods, such as peanut butter and items prepared with partially hydrogenated oil, margarine and vegetable oil. As well as all deep fried "junk" food. Read your labels!

Dairy

While kefir and some yogurts are acceptable, dairy is hard on the body. People who are lactose intolerant don't produce the lactase enzyme, which is required to break down lactose, a sugar found in milk, causing digestive issues whenever they consume dairy products. Milk is a common allergen that can trigger inflammation, stomach problems, skin rashes, hives and even breathing difficulties. It is crucial to confirm through an elimination diet if you are sensitive or intolerant to dairy/lactose. If you have an intolerance, it is best to remove it from your diet. If not, keep the quantities of dairy you consume as low as possible. Dairy is acid forming, inflammatory, and contains hormones and antibiotics.[4]

Dairy also contains casein and whey. Unlike lactose intolerance, casein and whey can cause an actual immune response and be considered a true allergy by promoting an IgE response from the immune system. And this immune response can cause inflammation.

Feedlot-Raised Meat

Animals who are fed grains like wheat, soy and corn are highly inflamed. Any meats bought from your local supermarket are grain and soy fed. These animals also gain excess fat and are injected with hormones and antibiotics. Always opt for organic, free-range meats from animals which have been fed natural diets.

Red and Processed Meat

Red meat contains a molecule that humans don't naturally produce called Neu5GC. Once you ingest this compound, your body develops antibodies which may trigger constant inflammatory responses. Reduce red meat consumption and replace with poultry, fish and lean cuts of red meat, once a week at most.

Alcohol

Regular consumption of alcohol causes irritation and inflammation to numerous organs, which can lead to cancer. Enjoying one or two glasses of wine a week is fine if your body tolerates it. If you are extremely inflamed, it is best to remove alcohol from your diet until such time that your inflammation has subsided. Then you can again enjoy the occasional social drink.

Refined Grains / Gluten

"Refined" products contain no fiber and have a high glycaemic index. They are everywhere: white rice, white flour, white bread, pasta, pastries, crisps, pizza, cakes, biscuits etc.

Dr Osborne calls himself the gluten free warrior. He is also the author of *No Grain No Pain*. He has done extensive work in the gluten free arena. In the video provided in the link, he highlights that ALL grains contain gluten.[5] This includes wheat, corn, rice, rye and quinoa. This video is almost an hour long, but worthwhile to watch.

He highlights that grains contain mycotoxins, gluten and glyphosate (a pesticide being used on grains). All three of these aspects can lead to health issues. Hence the importance of testing your sensitivity for all grains. He warns that some people may be more sensitive to rice gluten or corn gluten than wheat gluten.

We have discussed gluten at length. If you have an autoimmune disease, it is recommended that you **<u>completely</u>** remove gluten from your diet. Start with wheat (gluten). After that you can test your sensitivity to other gluten forms such as corn.

Removing gluten from your diet, could be the single most important action you can take to improve your health within a week.

Removing gluten means ALL gluten. Not only bread, bakes, pastries and pasta. Gluten is hidden in soup powders, bottled sauces, spices, beer, meats and processed foods. Dr Osborne posted a list of food ingredients on his website which could contain hidden gluten:

- MSG
- Modified food starch / wheat starch (found in most meats)
- Textured vegetable protein
- Hydrolyzed plant protein
- Hydrolyzed vegetable protein
- Hydrogenated Starch Hydrolysate
- Hydroxypropylated Starch
- Pregelatinized starch
- Vegetable gum
- Vegetable protein
- Extenders and binders
- Maltodextrin (wheat or corn based)
- Dextrin
- Maltose
- Non dairy creamer
- Seasonings (check labels)
- Natural flavours
- Smoke flavours
- Artificial flavours
- Natural colours
- Artificial colours
- Caramel colour and flavouring
- Soy sauce

- Dip mixes
- Dry sauce mixes
- Honey Hams – can be based with wheat starch in coating.
- Ice Cream & Frozen Yogurt – check all dairy. Cows are fed grains and many react to dairy for this reason. Grass fed dairy recommended (or avoid dairy altogether)
- Instant teas & coffees – cereal products may be included in the formulation
- Mayonnaise – check thickener and grain based vinegar ingredients
- Mustard – Mustard powder may contain gluten
- Oil, frying – Check for cross contamination or corn based oils
- Poultry and meats – Check out the flavourings and basting and inquire about meat glue
- Sour cream – May contain modified food starch of indeterminate source
- Dry roasted nuts & honey roasted nuts

     Your Greatest Wealth is your Health   94

• Stock cubes	• French fries in restaurants – Same oil may be used for wheat-containing items
• Candy may be dusted with wheat flour	• Gravies – check out thickening agent and liquid base
• Canned soups (Most are not acceptable)	• Vitamin supplements (different brands contain grain based ingredients – check the labels carefully)
• Cheese spreads & other processed cheese foods	• Baking powder (commonly contains grain – wheat or corn)
• Chocolate – may contain malt flavouring	
• Cold cuts, Wieners, Sausages – may have gluten due to cereal fillers	

This list is scary right?! This list will help you make better food choices. You would need to become conscious of food labels.[6]

Ty Bollinger, Co-Founder of Organixx, published an article where he highlights the top 10 causes of inflammation:[7]

1. Foods with a high glycemic (GI) index and added sugar. Chocolate is a major culprit

2. Trans Fats - contained in cakes, cookies, pies, margarine, crackers, biscuits, microwave popcorn, doughnuts, deep fried fast foods, frozen pizza etc

3. Saturated animals fats - dairy products, cheese, fatty meats, ice cream, cold meats

4. Excessive alcohol consumption

5. Celiac disease, and I would like to add non-celiac gluten sensitivity - bread is a major culprit!

6. Smoking

7. Chronic uncontrolled stress

8. Obesity

9. High ratio of omega 6 to omega 3 polyunsaturated fatty acids - a major culprit here is vegetable oils such as sunflower, soy, canola, peanut and mayonnaise and salad dressings[8]

10. Pollution and environmental toxins (see section 17)

Dr Tom O'Bryan says: "The fastest growing cells in your body are the cells in your intestines.[9] Every three to seven days, you have a completely new lining of your intestines. So, when you have toast for breakfast, you create tears in the lining of your intestines. Now larger molecules can get through. But it heals. You have a sandwich for lunch, and you tear your stomach lining. But it heals. You have pasta for dinner, and you tear your stomach lining. But it heals.[10] Every time you have an exposure to gluten, you get intestinal permeability within 36 hours, but it heals. But then one day you get intestinal permeability, and it doesn't heal. You cross an imaginary threshold, which you can't feel. Now you have pathogenic intestinal permeability and the whole cascade begins. Now should everyone give up gluten?

Being an opinion leader, I can't say that — it sounds too fanatical. **But I don't know why anyone would eat something that's definitely going to tear away at their body."** I have to agree with Dr O'Bryan.

You thus need to do an elimination diet to confirm which grains you may be sensitive to.

Do note that once you remove gluten from your diet, you may lack prebiotics. Wheat provides a major supply of prebiotics. When you go gluten free, it is important to increase your intake of prebiotic loaded veggies. This will be addressed in the next section: REPLACE.

Avoid high carbohydrate meals such as pasta, bread, porridge.[11]

Carbs are not bad for you. BAD CARBS are bad for you. In the Broken Brain Series, Dr Daniel Amen says: "Carbohydrates are really important—they're essential to life, but I want you to eat smart carbs—carbs that are loaded with nutrients and fiber, low-glycaemic carbs, which are carbs that don't raise your blood sugar. Think colourful. Carbs, berries, red bell peppers, orange bell peppers, and carrots, and kill the sugar before the sugar kills you."

Dr Christianson highlights three rules when eating carbs:[12]

Carb Rule 1 – Stick to eating good carbs

Dr Christianson says good carbs are the ones that burn the most slowly. The group of carbs that burns the fastest is fructose (as was also highlighted by Dr Mark Hyman). It is like gasoline. Fiber is slow like the campfire. Along with warding off disease, fiber is critical for good digestion and good immune function. Carbs that contain high levels of fiber and the least fructose include beans, intact whole grains, starchy vegetables and low-sugar fruits. Specific examples include black beans, pinto beans, beets, squash, sweet potatoes, blackberries and peaches.

Carb Rule 2 – Eat sufficient good carbs

Your personal need can vary based on your gender, the weight you are targeting, how stable your blood sugar is, how active you are and your gene patterns. That said, most people will do well somewhere between 1-2 cups per day total. (This will be the volume after cooking, not before.) Those seeking to lose weight can do well on the lower limit.[13]

Carb Rule 3 – Eat carbs at the right times

Your body responds to carbs differently based on the time of day you eat them. ***Eating them later in the day is better than earlier.*** When you eat your carbs later in the day, you will make them into energy instead of making them into fat.

Breakfast carbs could include ¼-½ cup of blackberries in a protein shake.[14] Lunch carbs could come from ½ cup of beans (legumes) or roasted beets on a salad with veggies and chicken. Dinner carbs could be from 1 cup of whole grain brown rice or cooked turnips in the context of a stir fry. Snacks could be nuts (raw nuts excluding peanuts) and low-carb veggies, like celery, cauliflower or broccoli. If you are not intolerant to nuts, they can have a major positive impact on your health. It has also been reported that nuts are high in antioxidants and could improve heart health. Raw almonds are particularly good.

These are really great guidelines by Dr Christianson.

For those with ulcers, some high carb foods may be required. Do consult your doctor, functional health practitioner, homeopath or an integrative health practitioner

Meals should consist of protein and healthy fats, with lots of fiber (fresh vegetables) from the anti-inflammatory list.

In the docuseries *Regain Your Brain*, it is emphasised in multiple episodes that consuming healthy fats is food for your brain. It is essential for good brain health.[15]

The top 5 healthy fats are avocados, butter from organic or grass fed sources, coconut oil, extra virgin olive oil and foods high in omega 3 such as wild caught salmon, walnuts and seeds (such as flaxseeds and chia seeds) and high quality cuts of meat such as grass fed beef.[16]

Let's consider what are good and what are bad carbs.

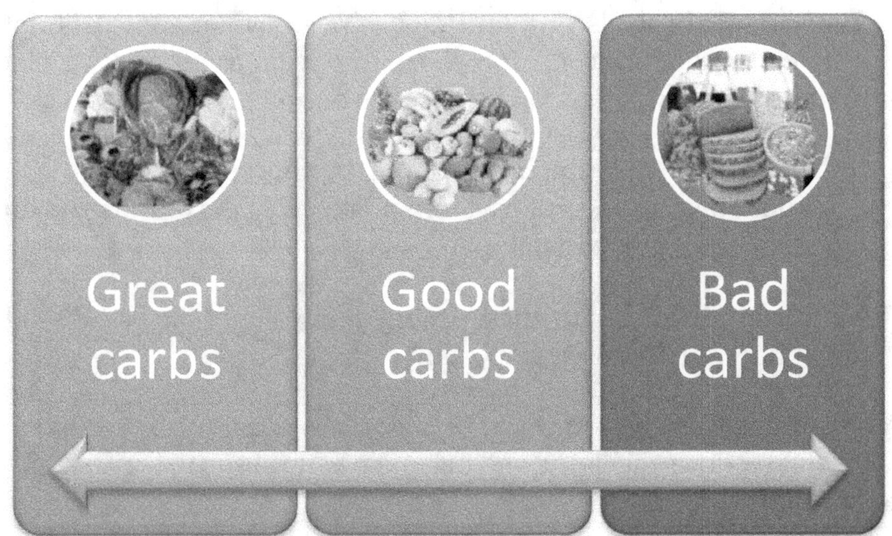

I guess you are a bit surprised. The media always refers to breads and cereals as carbs. Leafy greens, cruciferous veggies and berries contain the good carbs which you can freely enjoy!! The good carbs, your starchier veggies can be eaten in moderation. And sugary snacks, cold drinks, and breads and pastries should best be avoided.

Here is a list of food high in fiber.[17]

Food that are high in fiber		
Psyllium husks	Almonds	Blackberries
Chia seeds	Avocados	Brussel sprouts
Flaxseeds	Raspberries	

Just know that ALL VEGGIES contain a good solid amount of fiber. You cannot go wrong with veggies.[18]

Incorporate these into your diet, rather than using artificial fiber supplements.

Legumes and wheat also contain high levels of fiber. But it is not recommended that you consume wheat. And as far as legumes go, you need to first see if you have an intolerance or not.

Coconut flour is also high in fiber! If you are battling with constipation, take a spoon of psyllium husk on a glass of water on an empty stomach 1-3 times a day.

Fiber can be divided into three categories: soluble, insoluble and resistant fiber. All three are important.

Soluble fiber (dissolves in water) – reduces cholesterol, keeps blood sugar stable, slows digestion and helps the body absorb nutrients and keeps you full. Examples are:

- Nuts & Seeds
- Beans / Legumes: black, kidney and navy beans, lentils
- Fruits: citrus fruits, apples, pears, oranges, figs
- Veggies: Carrots, sweet potato, peas, avocado, brussel sprouts, asparagus,
- Psyllium husk
- Oats
- Blue berries, strawberries, dried figs

Insoluble fiber (does not dissolve in water) – increases bulk and prevents constipation, speed up food passing through the intestinal track and removes toxins. Examples are:

- Avocado
- Fruits with skin: Apple skin, Strawberries, dried figs, dried coconut, dried prunes and dates
- Lentils, brown rice, whole grains, wheat bran
- Flaxseed

- Nuts, pistachio nuts, almonds, red kidney beans, lima beans, chickpea
- Veggies with skin: Celery, zucchini, cabbage, beets, Brussel sprouts, cauliflower, bell peppers
- Fermented veggies – probiotics and digestive enzymes

Resistant fiber, also called resistant starch improves your metabolism and blood sugar while optimizing your gut flora to promote weight loss.[19] Resistant starch is not digested in the small intestine, hence its name. Instead, your gut bacteria processes it, creating beneficial molecules that promote balanced blood sugar and healthy gut flora. In other words, when you eat resistant starch, it "resists" digestion and does not spike blood sugar or insulin. Examples are:

- Legumes
- Green bananas
- Raw potato starch – bought in powder form
- Cooked and cooled potatoes – they should not be reheated!

Remove all processed foods, preserved foods and chemical enhanced foods. Go for whole foods!

Aspartame and MSG are two common food additives that can trigger inflammation responses. Try and omit these completely from the diet. **Artificial food additives, preservatives, colourants, flavourants wreak havoc in your body. All processed foods, preserved foods and chemical enhanced foods should be avoided at all cost.**

I cannot emphasize just how important it is to not touch processed foods. The obvious culprits are sausages, viennas, cold meats, or processed meats in tins, processed vegetables in tins. Unfortunately, it does not stop there.

Any foods that are genetically modified (GMO), containing preservatives or are chemically enhanced should be avoided.

How do you know foods are processed or modified. The best way is to start reading labels. If there is anything on a label which you can't pronounce, it is highly likely not to be good for you. It also goes for sugar free and gluten free products. A lot of these products sold as healthy are highly processed. It is best to prepare your own gluten free snacks.

Start reading food labels!

A whole food diet means natural, organic foods with no hormones, pesticides, preservatives, colourants etc. It includes fresh meats, vegetables, fruits and salads.

The best option is to go organic. Why is it important to go organic? Besides the fact that most meats are injected with growth hormones, these animals also eat food that has been sprayed by pesticides. Grass fed cattle that are allowed to range freely on open pastures do not carry this risk. The safest meat to eat is grass fed, grass finished livestock.

Same goes for vegetables, fruits and salads. For a great selection of organic foods that can be ordered online, check this out https://www.faithful-to-nature.co.za/. or visit Jacksons Real Food Market http://jacksonsrealfoodmarket.co.za. Jackson now has a store in Bryanston, and one in Kyalami.

If you can't go 100% organic day one, at least start eating whole foods. These foods are still loaded with dense nutrients that will have a major impact on your health!

Pesticides, which are any substance intended to prevent or destroy pests, are used to protect food from bacteria, weeds, mould, insects and rodents.[20] It has been found that pesticides damage the gut wall.[21]

According to the Environmental Protection Agency, pesticides can be harmful to people, animals or the environment because they are designed to kill or harm living organisms. Because of this, pesticide residue on the foods you eat can have an effect on your health.

Paula Owens says: "Serious health hazards have been linked to GMOs, pesticides, herbicides and glyphosate including infertility, immune problems, accelerated aging, significant inflammation, faulty insulin regulation, autoimmune disease, and changes in major organs and the gastrointestinal system." She indicates that glyphosate is the active ingredient in Roundup herbicide. Exposure to glyphosate is partially to blame for rising rates of autism, neurological disorders and chronic diseases.[22]

Zen Honeycutt, in the Addiction Summit indicates that in the latter part of the 90s our food supply was changed - GMOs or genetically modified organisms were introduced.

There are three types of GMOs:

1. Round Up Ready Crops - Crops such as soy, corn, wheat had their DNA changed to withstand the herbicide Round Up (which contains Glyphosate). The Round Up absorbs in the plants and no matter how well we wash our fruits/veggies, we can't get rid of it...it destroys our beneficial gut bacteria.

2. The second type had a pesticide (BT Toxin) genetically engineered into the plant - if a bug eats this plant (with the BT Toxin), it dies. It destroys the bug's gut and ultimately their tummies explode. Unfortunately the same happens to our guts/tummy lining!

3. Desired Trait GMO - here crops are engineered to contain a specific trait such as more Vit A, or an apple that does not brown, redder tomatoes etc.

Paula Owens quotes the following sources of genetically modified organisms (GMOs), Pesticides and Glyphosate:[23]

- 90% or more of ALL soybeans and soy-derived ingredients, rice, corn (flours, syrups and sweeteners), canola and cottonseed oils, and sugar beets grown in the U.S. are genetically modified! About 55 percent of the sugar produced in the U.S. comes from sugar beets, 95 percent of which have been genetically engineered.
- GMOs are found in ALL processed foods, some fruits and vegetables, and in alarming quantities in animal feed and pet food. **If you eat processed foods and non-organic conventional animal protein, you're consuming glyphosate residues.**
- **All grains are sprayed with Round Up (glyphosate**). Besides wheat and grains, glyphosate is applied on barley, oats, canola, sunflower, flax, peas, lentils, dry beans and sugar cane.
- Dairy products from cows injected with rbGM, a Genetically Modified (GM) hormone
- Meat and eggs from animals that have eaten GM feed (i.e. corn, soy, alfalfa).
- Food additives, artificial sweeteners, flavourings and processing agents, and rennet used to make hard cheeses
- Flaxseed oil and vegetable oils (corn, soybean, canola, safflower, rapeseed, cottonseed).
- Honey and bee pollen that may have GM sources of pollen.
- Non-food items that may contain GM ingredients include personal care products, aspartame found in some supplements, children's vitamins, over the counter medications and laxatives.
- Other items containing GMOs include infant formula, pet food, peanut butter, conventional factory-farmed animal protein, candy, beer, alcohol, salad dressing, coffee, bread, cereals, crackers, canned soup, cookies, chocolate, chewing gum, fried food, chips, juice, margarine, mayonnaise, hamburgers, veggie burgers, hotdogs, ice cream, frozen yogurt, tofu, soy sauce, soy cheese, tomato sauce, some protein powders, baking powder, vanilla, sugar, flour and pasta.

     Your Greatest Wealth is your Health

Can you see the similarity between this list and the list by Dr Osborne on foods containing gluten? The above information makes one think. Hence the importance of going whole foods and going organic.

For ultimate health, going organic is the way!

The Environmental Working Group has done research to highlight the dirty dozen to indicate which foods should be eaten as organic at all cost. Their Clean 15 can be eaten non-organic as they have a lesser absorption of herbicides and pesticides.

EWG's 2018 Dirty 12		
Strawberries	Peaches	Potatoes
Spinach	Cherries	Sweet bell peppers
Nectarines	Pears	
Apples	Tomatoes	
Grapes	Celery	

EWG's 2018 Clean 15		
Avocados	Sweet peas	Honeydews
Sweet corn	Papayas	Kiwis
Pineapples	Asparagus	Cantaloupes
Cabbages	Mangoes	Cauliflower
Onions	Eggplants	Broccoli

You can see that most baked goods are also considered to be processed or modified. No baked goods should be eaten unless you have baked it yourself or have a trusted source.[24]

Do note that all bottled sauces contain preservatives, food enhancers, colourants and or gluten. **Rather make your own.**

This may sound like a bit much, but changing your diet to simple, natural, organic whole foods can have a massive impact on your health.

Fizzy drinks

Stop drinking all carbonated drinks. It contains high levels of sugar, phosphoric acid, artificial sweeteners and caffeine which are all bad for your health. Do note, if you have an ulcer, carbonated drinks should be avoided at all cost! It is not worth it.[25]

Any foods you may have an intolerance for

This is a really important message to follow. Stop and listen: Do you constantly have headaches or feel tired? Sometimes, you may develop an allergy to a food and not even know it. Coffee, certain vegetables, cheese... there might be a trigger you aren't even aware of.

Many food intolerances develop because people do not eat enough variety.

Eating too much of the same food can lead to an intolerance. I believe that many of the current protein diets lead to food intolerances. People overeat cheese and biltong, and soon they can't eat it anymore.

It may be good time to talk about the Keto Diet at this point. The Keto Diet has huge benefits if approached correctly. The Keto Diet promotes eating low carb and high fat. If the fats are limited to healthy fats such as avocados, coconut, nuts etc, this diet will have amazing anti-inflammatory effects. But if the focus is on bad fats such as cream cheese, cream etc, you will initially lose weight, but soon these inflammatory foods will have the opposite effect.

My personal view is that there is no one diet for anyone.

Diet is something you need to personalise for yourself, based on your blood type, your food intolerances and any health conditions you may have.

Try and take a few foods out to see how you feel and slowly incorporate them back in to see if there might be a hidden culprit lurking in your diet![26]

Foods most people have intolerance for are:

- Cow's milk / dairy products
- Eggs
- Peanuts
- Tree nuts
- Grains (all foods/grains with gluten)
- Fish / Shellfish
- Soybeans
- Red meat
- Corn
- Legumes (especially an issue for people with autoimmune diseases) – that said, if soaked well over night before cooking it, it should have no or a lesser effect.
- Night shade vegetables (it is especially an issue for people with autoimmune diseases)
  o Tomatoes
  o Paprika
  o Cayenne pepper
  o Capsicum
  o White potatoes
  o Eggplant
  o Goji berries
  o Peppers (red, green, yellow)
  o Sorrel
  o Gooseberries
  o Ground cherries
  o Tobacco

Many people are intolerant to dairy products. Some people seem to be sensitive to milk and cheese but can tolerate plain yogurt. Others can cope with any dairy. If you fit in this category, rather avoid dairy, you will very soon see the health benefits.

Should you be able to tolerate cheese, do note that all cheeses are not equal. **Your healthier versions are feta cheese, cottage cheese and goats milk cheese.** Cheese that is processed, has added sugar and hormones, and is not the way to go. This includes cheeses such as cream cheese. [27]

Eating good quality meat that is hormone free is very important! Meat often contains gluten. Do yourself and favour and read the food labels on meat. Grass fed, organic, free range meats that are gluten free is the best option! I personally do not respond well to red meat. I eat red meat once a week. The rest of the time I eat chicken or fish, or other good sources of protein such as seeds, nuts and legumes.

If you have an autoimmune disease, do take the legumes and night shades seriously! First make sure you do not have an intolerance.[28] Above is a list of night shade vegetables courtesy of Dr Axe. Should you not have an intolerance, these are really good for you. As mentioned earlier, by soaking legumes over night you may remove the issue. I find that I can eat legumes if soaked well, and night shades in moderation.

You will need to do an elimination diet to confirm if you are intolerant to any of the above. Remove all from your diet for at least 2 weeks, then reintroduce one at a time and see if you have any reaction. Remember, some foods have a delayed reaction. Wait at least 5 days to see if you experience any symptoms.

Avoid pesticides

All forms of toxic poison should be avoided at all cost. Natural alternatives do exist. Here is a list of herbal remedies.[29]

- Ants – Cinnamon or corn starch
- Bugs – Combine garlic and mint with cayenne pepper and non-toxic dishwashing liquid
- Spiders and fish moths – Peppermint oil (10-15 drops in a spray bottle with water)
- Flies and mosquitos – a few drops of citronella oil mixed with coconut oil or a citronella plant[30]

Always remember to buy pure essential oils. If they are loaded with artificial fragrance, they become toxic. Check your labels.

In South Africa, a fantastic product is available called BioKill. It is available from PnP stores and Builders Warehouse countrywide.[31]

On the Greenmedinfo website, you can find extensive research on pesticides that may interest you.

Remove Parasites

Removing parasites from the body is an important step toward greater health.[32]

Dr Jay Davidson recommends treating parasites with Mimosa Pudica Seed Extract. It can be ordered https://www.mountainfresh.co.uk/product/putri-malu-mimosa-pudica-sensitive-plant-capsules/.

If you are interested, check out the video by Dr Alan Christianson where he unpacks the various types of parasites and how they can be treated.[33]

Untreated parasites and infections can seriously affect your health. Speak to your functional medicine practitioner. Dr Ann Louise

Gittleman indicates that way of preventing parasites are: cook your food well, avoid eating salads at salad bars, do not use a microwave as the primary way to cook food and wash your salads well. She says that sugar and dairy feeds parasites.[34]

Make sure to work with your functional health practitioner, homeopath or an integrative health practitioner to address parasites.

I have great news though! What you eat can either feed parasites or fight parasites. Sugar is the biggest culprit that feeds parasites. Two great strategies to fight parasites are doing intermittent fasting (which is unpacked later in this book) and eating anti-parasitic herbs and foods. Great options include coconut oil, garlic, cucumber seeds, papaya, clove, raw pumpkin seeds, turmeric, ginger, cayenne and black walnut. Add these to your diet on a regular basis.

Avoid all environmental toxins
(Refer to SECTION 17 ON ENVIRONMENTAL TOXINS)

- BPA in plastics
- Foil
- Tap water
- Toxic personal care products
  - Body and facial creams
  - Make-up
  - Soaps, body washes, shower gels
  - Hair products (shampoo, conditioner, hair spray, hair mask, anti-frizz etc)
  - Nail products
  - Perfume / deodorant
  - Sun screen
- Toxic cleaning chemicals
  - Kitchen and bathroom cleaner
  - Tile cleaner

- o Furniture polish
  - o Laundry detergent
  - o Oven cleaner
  - o Stain remover
  - o Window cleaner
- Air fresheners
- Hand sanitisers
- Pesticides / Insect repellents

There are so many great stores and online stores where one can get non-toxic alternatives. My favourites are:

- Faithful to Nature[35]
- Jacksons Real Food Market[36]
- Wellness Warehouse[37]

I make my own home-made household cleaners and personal care products. A fantastic go-to product is Castile soap, which is a Pure-Simple product. I find it is quite expensive to buy green products. For me it is far more cost effective to make them myself.

When you go to your local pharmacy, take care to read labels. Many products are sold as natural, but still contain preservatives, fragrances, flavouring and parabens which are endocrine disrupters.

Avoid leftovers

Rules relating to leftovers:[38]

1. Leftovers should only be heated up once and only once!
2. Food should be refrigerated within 2 hours of being cooked. Leftovers should be eaten within 2 days.
3. Keep leftovers covered.

4. Contain it wisely, preferably in a glass container. Do not package warm food in plastic containers.

Olivia Lerche reports that the Food Standards Agency says that uncooked rice can contain spores of bacteria that can cause food poisoning.[39] When the rice is cooked, the spores can survive. Then, if the rice is left standing at room temperature, the spores will multiply and may produce poisons that cause vomiting or diarrhoea. Reheating the rice won't get rid of these poisons. This means that the longer cooked rice is left at room temperature, the more likely it is that poisons produced could stop the rice being safe to eat. It's best to serve rice when it has just been cooked.

Remove antacids, proton pump inhibitors (PPIs) and antibiotics

These medicines should only be used when really needed. Using any of these on a chronic basis will destroy your gut bacteria. Check in with your functional medicine expert or integrative health practitioner for advice.

Remove / manage emotional toxins

Removing or at the very least dealing with emotional stress or toxins, including toxic thoughts, is fundamental to health! In Section 16, Rebalance Your Life, we will cover this in detail.

Remove infections and parasites

As was mentioned before, infections and parasites can wreak havoc on your body. Speak to your functional medicine practitioner to help you identify hidden infections, this could include speaking to a biological dentist to confirm if you do not have infections in your cavities. And do a parasite cleanse every 6 months. Speak to your local health shop for the best local product at your disposal.

The best way to tackle the REMOVE stage, is to first remove the BIG culprits that you suspect to be your issue. For most people these are gluten, sugar and dairy. Tackle them one at a time. If you make too many changes at once you may not be able to recognise which of these changes have a positive impact on your health.

Reality is that we will always be exposed to toxins in our foods and our environment. You need to take control over what you have control of. You cannot control everything. **The beauty is that a single change, such as removing gluten, can have a MASSIVE impact on your health.** Take it one step at a time. Remove the big culprits and see what an amazing effect it has on your body. That would be your motivation to tackle the next culprit. It took me three years to get where I am. Given you now know what to do, it need not take you three years, but it also does not have to take a month. **Allow your body to enjoy the changes and to tell you how it feels about these changes.**

Too many changes at once will prevent you from identifying the real culprits making you ill.

Looking back, I cherish the time it took to get where I am today.

Sources of References in Section 12

1. http://realfoodcon.com/dr-tom-obryan/
2. https://brokenbrain.com/
3. https://draxe.com/what-sugar-does-to-your-brain/
4. https://www.mindbodygreen.com/0-8646/the-dangers-of-dairy.html
5. https://www.youtube.com/watch?v=Tz9-7_mlMvE
6. https://www.glutenfreesociety.org/guidelines-for-avoiding-gluten-unsafe-ingredients-for-gluten-sensitivity/#ySoMDIJ3eLJI1lql.99

7. https://organixx.com/what-causes-inflammation/?gl=5ae0a514210d2a5d36b53949&mpweb=693-6750665-742333721

8. http://certifiedglutenpractitioner.com/videos/

9. https://www.ncbi.nlm.nih.gov/pubmed/25701700?inf_contact_key=f3ec61ad653a418ff8e4e40df76a2d5e72426aa502d0e1a8b07dc27089e56679

10. http://www.missionheirloom.com/blog/2016/1/29/dr-tom-obryan

11. https://brokenbrain.com/

12. https://www.huffingtonpost.com/alan-christianson/are-carbs-evilpart-two_b_6295764.html

13. http://www.greenmedinfo.com/blog/eating-more-antioxidant-rich-nuts-improves-heart-health

14. http://www.greenmedinfo.com/blog/what-15-almonds-day-can-do-you

15. https://regainyourbrain.awakeningfromalzheimers.com/new-episode

16. http://healthintegrations.com/blog/2015/08/22/the-5-best-healthy-fats-for-your-body---by-dr-axe

17. https://low-carb-support.com/low-carb-high-fibre/

18. https://www.pegym.com/nutrition/is-there-such-a-thing-as-good-carbs

19. https://www.todaysdietitian.com/newarchives/090112p22.shtml

20. https://www.livestrong.com/article/505005-how-to-soak-vegetables-fruit-in-sea-salt-water-to-remove-pesticides/

21. http://www.nourishingplot.com/2014/02/11/foods-act-as-pesticides-within-leaky-gut-patients/

22. https://theaddictionsummit.com/expert/zen-honeycutt/

23. https://paulaowens.com/gmos-pesticides-glyphosate/

24. https://geneticliteracyproject.org/2018/04/11/viewpoint-environmental-working-groups-dirty-dozen-list-highlights-meaningless-distinctions-between-organic-and-conventional-foods/

25. https://wellnessmama.com/379/reasons-to-avoid-soda/

26. http://www.chicagonow.com/clean-convenient-cuisine/2010/09/best-and-worst-top-10-most-inflammatory-and-anti-inflammatory-foods/

27. https://draxe.com/healthiest-cheese/.

28. http://www.diagnosisdiet.com/nightshades/
29. http://www.sheknows.com/home-and-gardening/articles/1101763/alternatives-to-pesticides
30. https://www.builders.co.za/Garden-%26-Outdoor-Living/Garden/Pest-Control/Bio-Kill-Classic-(325ml)
31. http://www.greenmedinfo.com/toxic-ingredient/pesticides
32. http://drjaydavidson.com/removing-parasites-fix-lyme/
33. http://drchristianson.com/the-truth-about-parasites-avoiding-treating-and-defeating/?inf_contact_key=d0b46dc4257bb2e3c305754d6d841eca7ef9a3a8413b8a5ffa53e1e3056fcbe0
34. https://healthygutexperts.com/day-2/ann-louise-gittleman-3/
35. https://www.faithful-to-nature.co.za/
36. http://jacksonsrealfoodmarket.co.za
37. https://www.wellnesswarehouse.com/
38. https://nutritiouslife.com/live-consciously/rules-for-eating-leftovers/
39. https://www.express.co.uk/life-style/health/666554/reheating-rice-food-poisoning

Section 13
Replace

REPLACE INFLAMMATORY FOODS WITH ANTI-INFLAMMATORY FOODS

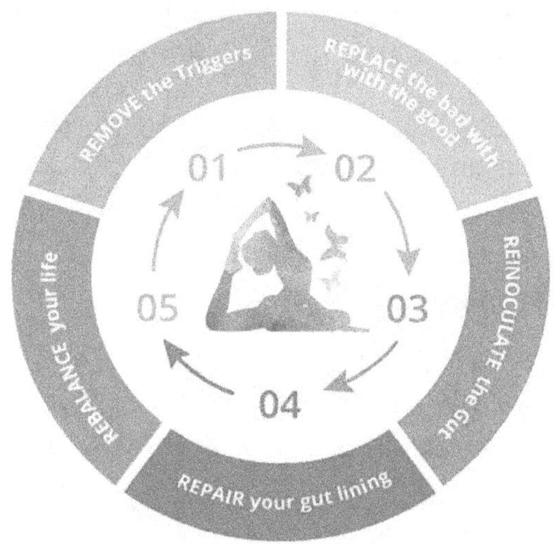

Time to add the good stuff

Replacing inflammatory foods with anti-inflammatory foods is a very important step in the process. By consuming anti-inflammatory foods, you will reduce the inflammation in your body at a pace that will amaze you!! This is one of the easiest steps in the programme. Removing inflammatory foods and toxins may take some time and may take some getting used to. But replacing the bad stuff with the good stuff will be easier. Remember what I told you in Section 11: It is all about changing habits.

Once you change bad habits into good ones, it becomes far easier!

> When it comes to changing eating habits, it is important to have a crutch.
>
> In changing your diet, you should take care not to let yourself feel deprived. Make sure from day 1 that you have access to nice meals that will inspire you.
>
> Prepare healthy snacks as alternatives to all the bad stuff. You can do it!

Let's consider a few great habits:

Stay hydrated by drinking purified water, at least 2 litres a day

- **When waking up, immediately drink 2 glasses of water**

  By drinking water upon waking up, you start you day by flushing toxins from your body

- **Drink a glass of water with each meal**

  Start cultivating those good habits

- **Do not only drink purified water, also use it for your coffee and tea and for cooking your meals.**

  It is so easy these days to have your water refilled. Get yourself a 25 liter can and refill while you are at the fuelling station (most fuelling stations now have water refill facilities).

- **Start using 1 teaspoon of <u>RAW</u> apple cider vinegar in a FULL glass of water on an empty stomach before meals**

  You should never exceed two table spoons a day. Rather start with a low doses. Drinking a lot of apple cider vinegar can damage your teeth, hurt your throat, and upset your stomach. Never drink undiluted apple cider vinegar. Also make sure you only use RAW apple cider vinegar. DO NOTE, some people are very sensitive to apple cider, if you note that your acid levels are raised or you are just not feeling well, rather cut down on your apple cider intake. If you feel a burning sensation in your tummy, rather do not use it, it is making you too acidic.

What does apple cider vinegar do? According to Dr Axe, taking RAW apple cider vinegar on an empty stomach has the following benefits:[1]

1. Decreases blood sugar
2. Supports weight loss, especially in conjunction with dietary changes[2]
3. Lowers cholesterol, in particular bad cholesterol
4. Improves skin health – texture, pigmentation and appearance
5. Reduces blood pressure – (it should be taken with care by anyone who has low blood sugar)
6. Relieves acid reflux symptoms as it introduces more acid in the digestive tract that prevents acid backflow[3]

Raw apple cider vinegar looks murky. You will very easily distinguish it from processed vinegar. Raw means it has not been filtered or pasteurised.[4]

On your journey, you are at some point or another likely to experience acid reflux.[5] In severe cases you feel like you are having a heart attack. Gastroesophageal reflux can cause chest pain and other symptoms that mimic those of a heart attack or angina, a crushing type of chest pain caused by decreased blood flow to the heart. It feels like someone is strapping a belt around your chest underneath your breasts and pulling it tight. Or that is how I felt! On my journey I twice rushed to the ER thinking I am having a heart attack. Both instances I had severe acid reflux. The message here once again is that you should listen to your body. If you make poor food choices, focusing on acidic foods, or just not eating enough alkaline foods, you could bring about these terrible symptoms. [6]

The answer lies in variety. Do not fall into the trap of eating too much of the same foods.

Follow an anti-inflammatory diet. Introduce foods such as:

- Raw Apple cider vinegar (no more than two table spoons a day!)
- Blue berries
- COCONUT (in all forms!)
- Turmeric
- Ginger
- Almonds
- Cabbage
- Cauliflower
- Brussel sprouts
- Flax seed
- Olive Oil
- Avocado
- Cinnamon
- Garlic
- Asparagus
- Sauerkraut
- Lemon (in moderation)
- Walnuts
- Chillies
- Cucumber
- Chai seeds
- Leafy greens such as spinach

> **Bombarding your body with a variety of anti-inflammatory foods will very quickly render results.**

Take note that you could have developed an intolerance for any of these foods, even though not highly likely. There is a chance. It is time to listen to your body! If you suspect a culprit, remove it from your diet for two weeks, reintroduce and see what happens.

We unknowingly eat so many inflammatory foods. As Dr Tom O'Bryan says, "It is adding fuel to the fire". If your gut is already so inflamed that your whole body is in pain, it is very important to avoid inflammatory foods at all cost.

Most people battle to make this adjustment. Remember you have to start somewhere. Start by removing the big culprits and introducing healthy alternatives that you enjoy. Be sure to avoid foods you have an intolerance for. We will talk more about this later.

Regularly eat a handful of organic blue berries

Put them in smoothies or eat them fresh or frozen as a snack. Their benefits include:[7]

- High in Antioxidants
- Help Fight Cancer
- Amp Up Weight Loss
- Boost Brain Health
- Alleviate Inflammation
- Support Digestion
- Promote Heart Health

Blue berries can also tend to be a bit acidic. If you tend to be more acidic, eat fewer blue berries, or perhaps every second day.

Regularly eat cruciferous veggies

Cruciferous vegetables (cabbage, spinach, cauliflower, broccoli and Brussel sprouts) should be eaten daily as it detoxes the liver.

Some people like myself can't eat raw cruciferous vegetables. If cooked, they do me the world of good. Again, listen to your body.

Unfortunately, even if you eat very healthy food, you still might experience bloating after your meal. For example, broccoli, cauliflower, beans, kale and even apples often cause intense bloating, even in otherwise healthy people. This is because of its high fiber content. You may need additional digestive enzymes to properly digest these foods. If you get bloated, first try adding digestive enzymes.

At the end of this section I will address FODMAP. If you react to healthy foods, do read the section on FODMAPs.

Eat enough, colourful veggies[8]

Dr Ann Hathaway in the Broken Brain docuseries says "When you look at your plate, we want two thirds of what you put into your body to be vegetables," She says "We want a variety of colours and a variety of types of vegetables, right? We want non-GMO and organic as much as possible, because pesticides and insecticides are potential toxins."

Replace your cooking oils with coconut oil, olive oil or avocado oil[9]

Coconut oil and grape seed oil can be used in a high heat scenario. Olive oil or avo oil should not be heated. Use over salads.

Hempseed oil is also a great choice, it contains the optimal ratio of Omega 3 and Omega 6. It should also not be heated.

Consume coconut in all forms[10]

Dr Mark Hyman dispels the myth that coconut oil is bad for you.

He says it raises HDL, the good cholesterol and lowers LDL, the bad cholesterol. It boosts metabolism and immune function, reverses insulin resistance and improves cognitive function. It is also antimicrobial and anti-fungal. My personal favourite is that it reduces inflammation. **Coconut flakes are delicious and a healthy snack.**

You must note that once you add healthy fats to your diet, your body may need time to get used to it. If you introduce too much too fast you will experience diarrhoea, nausea or acne breakout. Rather start slowly.[11]

Coconut oil can cause this reaction due to its effective anti-fungal, anti-bacterial and anti-viral properties. This may pass after just a few days of consistent use and gradually introducing it into the diet usually bypasses this.

A reaction known as die off, or a Herxheimer reaction, is thought to happen when toxins from dying pathogens (viruses, bacteria, parasites, candida, etc.) overload the body faster than it can clear them out. Hence symptoms such as nausea and vomiting.

Another possible side effect of eating too much fat too fast is the impact on your gall bladder. If at any time you get nauseous, cut back on your fats and visit your medical practitioner. Foods that can irritate your digestive system (if your gall bladder and or liver are battling to digest fats) include animal fats, onions, cheese, eggs and nuts.

Go for free range eggs

Eggs are really good for you if you do not have an intolerance. It has the perfect balance of amino acids. The nutrients in every egg you eat, however only come from the feed available to the chickens. Ingredients fed to the hens make a profound difference to the quality of each egg. Thus, go for free range.

Consume bone broth[12]

Bone broth is essential if you are in the process of healing your leaky gut. It improves your digestion, supports bone health and supports your immune system. There are various recipes you can find on the internet. The most basic recipe is using water, a little apple cider vinegar, and beef or chicken bones, and simmer in a slow cooker for 24 hours with some onion, celery, carrot, salt and pepper. I love adding garlic and ginger for taste. Once done, strain the bone broth, let it cool down, remove the fat layer and drink or use in food such as soups or stews. Start off with a quarter cup diluted with water and build up to a half cup diluted with water. Bone broth is very concentrated, it is important not to drink too much undiluted. If it hurts your stomach, dilute some more.

Replace table salt with natural herbs, spices and Himalayan salt

Too much sodium (salt) in your system results in your body retaining water. This puts an extra burden on the heart and blood vessels. In some people this may lead to high blood pressure. Having less sodium in your diet may help you lower or avoid high blood pressure. People with high blood pressure are more likely to develop heart disease or have a stroke.

Most of the sodium in our diet comes from adding it when food is prepared and from processed foods. Pay attention to food labels, because they indicate the amount of sodium in the product.

Herbs and certain spices have amazing health benefits. **When buying spices, look at the ingredients and avoid those that contain monosodium glutamate (MSG), a flavour enhancer and gluten.** Making a decision to avoid MSG and gluten in your diet is a wise choice. It does take a bit more planning and time in the kitchen to prepare food at home, using fresh, locally grown ingredients. Knowing that your food is pure and free of toxic additives, like MSG, will make it well worth it. In South Africa, Dis-Chem and Checkers have various natural ranges.

Try flavouring your food with herbs

Another great option is Himalayan salt. It is said to be the purest salt on earth. Himalayan salt is 85% sodium chloride, and the remainder contains 80+ minerals. These minerals can help your body balance your PH, regulate water content, remove toxins, help absorb nutrients, prevent muscle cramping, create balance and more. It is known for its pure taste and unique pinkish colour.

Use fresh, organic herbs and spices

Using fresh herbs and organic spices is really important. Most spices contain both gluten and MSG. Dr Axe provides a great list of all herbs and spice and their health benefits. [21]

My personal favourites are:

- Sage is great for naturally balancing hormones and supporting brain health.

- Turmeric is a must for daily consumption! It is amazing in treating inflammation.

- Cinnamon is a great antioxidant and helps balance blood sugar levels. Add a cinnamon stick to your cup of tea and see the difference!

- Basil has anti-inflammatory and antiviral properties.

- Garlic is a natural antibiotic.

- Cayenne can help with the absorption of other nutrients and help with pain management (It is a night shade. You should first make sure it is not a trigger for you).

- Mint and freshly grated ginger are great for adding flavour to water if you are not fond of drinking water.

- Oregano has antiviral, antibacterial, anticancer and antibiotic properties.

Sage, basil, mint, oregano or ginger can easily be added to a smoothie.

Meal combinations should include protein, healthy oils and fiber

Make sure meals contain a protein (for example fish, chicken, nuts (not peanuts) or pure protein powder), with healthy oils (for example avo, olive oil, coconut, wild caught salmon, olives, nuts and seeds) and fiber (vegetables). Remember to eat cruciferous veggies. (If you respond negatively to raw veggies, make sure to cook them).

Dr Mark Hyman, in his new book: **FOOD, What the heck should I eat?** says "if we don't eat adequate protein at every meal, our brains can't work. We will be sluggish, foggy, anxious, unfocused, tired, and depressed.". Remember protein does not necessarily mean meat, it could be nuts, seeds or legumes.[13]

Do remember, healthy fats, just like bad fats, still need to be digested. Hence the need for digestive enzymes. Do not eat too many fats as it could lead to gall bladder disfunction. Should you feel nauseous after a fatty meal, cut back on your fats and increase your digestive enzyme intake.

Add honey and papaya to your diet (in moderation)

Raw honey, papaya, raw pineapple and avocado are loaded with digestive enzymes. This is especially helpful for those of you who suffer from constipation. Most fruits are high in enzymes. Knowing that fruit sugar should be avoided in excess, my recommendation is that one eats at least one fruit a day.

Tips to naturally increase your liver's bile production[19]

If you add healthy fats to you diet, these tips become very important advice.

- Drink a glass of water with lemon upon awakening
- Avoid eating sugars and processed foods
- Consume bitter foods

- Eat garlic, onions, and carrots
- Drink tea made from dandelion, peppermint, green tea, or ginger
- Drink buttermilk and eat plain, unsweetened yogurt

Regularly eat home-made apple sauce[14]

Dr Tom O'Bryan indicates that home-made apple sauce can help heal a leaky gut.

Apple sauce can be made at home, use organic apples. Put 5 apples in a saucepan filling it up with filtered water to about a third. Add some cinnamon and raisons. Boil it until the apples become shiny. This means it is releasing pectin, which feeds the good bacteria in the tummy and supports your microbiome. He recommends eating a small bowl twice a day for a week...and every now and again after.

Cook your food in filtered water

Try not to cook your food in tap water. Rather be safe and use filtered water.[20]

Eat foods that enhance hydrochloric acid production

Hydrochloric acid helps your body digest food and in particular proteins. Examples include lemons, limes, apple cider vinegar, papaya, and high-quality salt (Himalayan).

Introduce as many anti-inflammatory foods to your diet as possible!

It is crucial to realise that people differ, and we all have different medical conditions and food intolerances. You have to take this into consideration when embarking on this journey. Even though all the foods listed in this section are good for you, some may not work for you!

You need to remove all food triggers that your body is reacting to, regardless if they may be anti-inflammatory. After three months of strictly following these guidelines, you can slowly reintroduce these foods one at a time and consider whether to add it back to your diet if you do not react to them.

Listen to your body!

Here is a great list of foods that are anti-inflammatory:[15]

ANTI-INFLAMMATORY FOODS	
Almonds	Walnuts
Cabbage	Chilies
Flax seeds	Blueberries
Olive Oil	Turmeric
Avocado	Ginger
Cinnamon	Brussel sprouts
Garlic	Coconut
Asparagus	Cucumber
Sauerkraut	Chia seeds
Walnuts	Raw apple cider vinegar
Lemon	Leafy greens
Wild Alaskan salmon	Green tea
Sweet potato	All berries

Load up on these in your diet and see the positive effect it has on your body.

Removing the inflammatory foods and adding these anti-inflammatory foods will change your life forever!

Should you have a peptic ulcer, consider the following[16]:

- Avoid all coffee and other sources of caffeine, including decaffeinated coffee, as well as alcohol and tobacco.

- Avoid milk and milk products as well, they increase acid secretion. Eat smaller amounts of foods more frequently.

- One of the most common symptoms of an ulcer is a burning sensation that often feels worse between meals. Milk and other dairy products, such as yogurt, coat the lining of the stomach. Because this seems to sooth the ulcer, many believe that drinking milk is one way to help cure an ulcer. On the contrary, milk stimulates the stomach to increase acid production, leading to an increase in ulcer irritation. If you have an ulcer, you should refrain from drinking milk and eating other dairy products as it can delay the healing of your ulcer.

Here are the top foods to consume as part of an ulcer diet for fast relief:

- Consume small meals – Eat several meals per day to reduce the burden on the digestive system and relieve ulcer symptoms.

- Enjoy high fiber foods – An increase in fiber can repair ulcers, aim for 30 grams per day. Eating a diet rich in fiber promotes a healthy digestive tract and can help reduce the risk of developing an ulcer and promotes healing of an active ulcer. To consume a high fiber diet, eat plenty of fruits and vegetables.

- Eat lots of green leafy vegetables – Green leafy vegetables provide Vitamin K that can help repair damage caused by too much stomach acid.

- Drink cabbage juice – It has been shown to heal ulcers. It can be diluted with some carrot juice for additional benefits.

- Eat plenty fermented foods. Good bacteria in the gut can help prevent H. pylori infection. Add kimchi, kefir, or unsweetened plain yogurt to your diet.

- Foods to avoid if you have an ulcer:[17]

- Refined wheat and dairy are all very inflammatory and should be avoided[18]

- Spicy foods can irritate ulcers. The link between spicy foods and ulcers is still not clear and the reaction from one patient to another is never the same. Some patients suffering from a peptic ulcer find their symptom of pain worsens after eating a meal containing spicy foods. The foods most likely to affect your ulcer include those with significant amounts of black pepper, chili powder, mustard seed or nutmeg. If you experience increased discomfort following a meal that contains a specific type of spice, avoid those spicy foods until your ulcer has had a chance to heal.

- Caffeine – Coffee and certain teas can make ulcers worse. Doctors classify caffeine as a stimulant because it stimulates the nervous system making you more alert and aware. Caffeine also stimulates acid production in the stomach and can, therefore, irritate your ulcer symptoms. To promote ulcer healing, refrain from eating and drinking foods and beverages that contain caffeine such as coffee and chocolates.

- Alcohol may actually trigger ulcers.

- Any potential food you have an allergy or intolerance for – Food allergies can cause ulcers or make them worse.

- Sugar is bad at its best! It can feed bad bacteria and make ulcers worse.

Once you have followed the anti-inflammatory diet for a few weeks, the inflammation in your body should slowly get under control. Once this happens, you could again enjoy some of these if you do not have a food intolerance. But until such time, give your digestion a break and allow the fire to die down.

As for the anti-inflammatory foods, you should keep on eating these for the rest of your life.

Foods I am really fond of are cabbage, cauliflower, coconut (in all forms), brussel sprouts, spinach and broccoli. These veggies are liver cleansing. By eating these at least twice a day, you keep your liver in good condition, and continuously support your liver to get rid of all the nasties. Another great addition to your diet is blue berries ... they are high in antioxidants.

But what if these healthy foods affect you on a bad way?

Be aware of FODMAPs and how they may impact your body[61]

FODMAPs is an acronym for "fermentable oligosaccharides, disaccharides, monosaccharides and polyols." These are specific types of sugars such as fructose, lactose, fructans and galactans that are found in carbohydrate foods such as certain vegetables, fruits, grains and dairy milk. FODMAPs are short-chained carbohydrates that are fermentable and can be poorly absorbed in the gut.

For a high percentage of people with IBS, reducing consumption of FODMAPs has been shown to help take the burden off the digestive system and improve symptoms. It is important to restrict food sources (primarily carbohydrates) that feed harmful bacteria in the gut.

Lifestyle changes and habits that can help manage IBS symptoms, especially exercise, getting enough sleep and stress management. Below is a table that can help guide you with what to eat and what to avoid if you are sensitive to FODMAPs.

Avoid	Limit	Enjoy!
Vegetables	**Vegetables**	**Vegetables**
Artichoke	Beets	Bamboo shoots
Asparagus	Broccoli	Carrots
Cauliflower	Butternut	Chives
Garlic	Pumpkin	Cucumbers
Green peas	Cabbage	Fresh herbs
Leek	Brussel sprout	Lettuce and salad greens
Mushrooms	Peas	Potatoes – cooked and cooled e.g. potato salad
Onion	Corn cob	Spinach
Sugar snap peas	Sweet potatoes	Zucchini / zucchini spaghetti
Leeks	Green peas	Tomato
	Asparagus	Spring onion – green part only
	Artichoke hearts (canned)	Gem Squash
	Celery	
Fruits	**Fruits**	**Fruits**
Apples	Avocado	Banana
Apple juice	Cherries	Berries
Cherries	Grapefruit	Grapes
Dried fruit	Shredded coconut	Kiwi
Mango		Orange
Nectarines		Pineapple
Peaches		Lemon
Tinned fruit		Lime
Fruit juice		Pawpaw
Honey		Strawberry
Pears		Lemon
Plums		Lime
Watermelon		Mandarin
Prune		Orange
		Passion fruit
		Pineapple

Avoid	Limit	Enjoy!
Dairy & Milk Cow's milk Goat's milk Custard Evaporated milk Ice cream Soy milk Sweetened condensed milk Yogurt Soft cheeses		**Dairy & Milk** Almond milk, coconut milk, rice milk Raw hard cheese (cheddar, parmesan) Lactose free yogurt
Protein Sources All processed meats Most legumes: baked beans, chickpea, lentil, red kidney bean		**Protein Sources** Eggs Grass-fed beef Grass-fed lamb Wild-caught fish Free-range chicken Free-range turkey Bone broth
Grains, Breads and Cereals Wheat Rye Barley Couscous Biscuits (salt or sweet) All cereals GMO corn flour products		**Grains, Breads and Cereals** Gluten free bread Gluten free oats Gluten free pasta

     Your Greatest Wealth is your Health

Avoid	Limit	Enjoy!
Sweetners High fructose corn syrup (in all processed foods! Read your labels) Sugar Honey		**Sweetners** Maple syrup
Nuts & Seeds Cashews Pistachios	**Nuts & Seeds** Almonds Hazel nuts	**Nuts & Seeds** Preferably sprouted or nut butters: Macadamia Pecans Pumpkin seeds Walnuts
		Seasonings & Condiments Coconut Oil Avocado Oil Grass fed butter Mayonnaise Herbs and gluten free spices Mustard Olives Vinegar

It's important to note that this list does not cover all foods that can and can't be eaten on the low FODMAP diet. You need to listen to your body!

Be aware of what you eat and how it affects your liver. I have a concern with people taking a ton of liver detox tablets but maintaining a diet which clogs the liver. It is time to act. You will feel the difference in no time! Decide today!

 Your Greatest Wealth is your Health 133

At this point I want to encourage you! If you experience fear that you won't get it right, and that you almost feel you do not want to eat anything as a result of your fear, just remember that God masterfully created the human body to not only cleanse itself, but also to protect and heal itself. All you need to do is your part (what is in your control), one step at a time, one day at a time, reduce your toxic load.

The easiest way to approach this section is by eating great variety of vegetables of different colours! The key is moderation and variety!

Too much of anything is not good for you!! The last thing you want to do it only eat one of two apparently good foods, and it ends up doing you harm because you eat too much of it.

To simplify your choices, go to the supermarket, and buy a mix of veggies of different colours, and eat those. If at first, these are not organic, it is still better than not eating veggies! As you grow into your new habits, you can consider growing your own veggies in your garden or buying organic from your farmers market. Just start somewhere.

Cruciferous veggies are amazing!! They will help you detox and you will feel the difference. Just start eating them. **And remember, add colour to your diet!** And remember to add extra water intake to your daily routine.

I want to remind you, a single change in your diet can change your world and your health.

The best bit of advice I can give you is to not buy the culprits. Stock your fridge with the good stuff.

And experiment with great recipes that are gluten free, or perhaps sugar or dairy free. There is so much available on the internet. In Section 18, I provide you with some ideas. Check out the snack ideas!!

If there is one thing I have learnt over the last three years, we all need a crutch. That crutch is a delicious recipe of a snack that is high in protein and healthy fats but tastes just as nice as your favourite sweet or snack.

Sources of References in Section 13

1. https://www.webmd.com/diet/apple-cider-vinegar-and-your-health
2. https://www.livestrong.com/article/237921-how-to-lose-weight-as-you-sleep-with-apple-cider-vinegar/
3. https://draxe.com/apple-cider-vinegar-uses/
4. https://www.faithful-to-nature.co.za/blog/need-know-buying-apple-cider-vinegar/
5. https://www.essence.com/lifestyle/health-wellness/signs-chest-pain-not-heart-attack#1094332
6. https://draxe.com/acid-reflux-symptoms/
7. https://draxe.com/health-benefits-blueberries/
8. https://brokenbrain.com/
9. http://www.zliving.com/health/natural-remedies/9-health-benefits-of-hemp-oil-that-you-should-know-2467/
10. www.drhyman.com/blog/2017/06/cocnut-oil/
11. https://www.coconutmybody.com.au/blogs/news/11038901-why-do-i-feel-sick-eating-coconut-oil/
12. https://blog.paleohacks.com/bone-broth-recipe/#
13. www.foodthebook.com
14. https://healthygutexperts.com/day-1/drtom/
15. https://healthyblenderrecipes.com
16. https://www.drweil.com/health-wellness/body-mind-spirit/gastrointestinal/peptic-ulcer-disease/
17. https://draxe.com/ulcer-symptoms-diet-natural-remedies/
18. https://www.livestrong.com/article/347146-what-to-eat-not-to-eat-when-you-have-an-ulcer/
19. https://www.belmarrahealth.com/bile-function-liver-foods-help-increase-bile-production/

20. http://www.onegreenplanet.org/natural-health/tips-to-improve-stomach-acid-levels-needed-for-good-digestion/

21. https://draxe.com/section/natural-remedies/herbs-spices/

22. https://www.healthline.com/nutrition/fodmaps#section1

Section 14

Reinoculate

REINOCULATE – ADD BACK GOOD BACTERIA INTO YOUR TUMMY

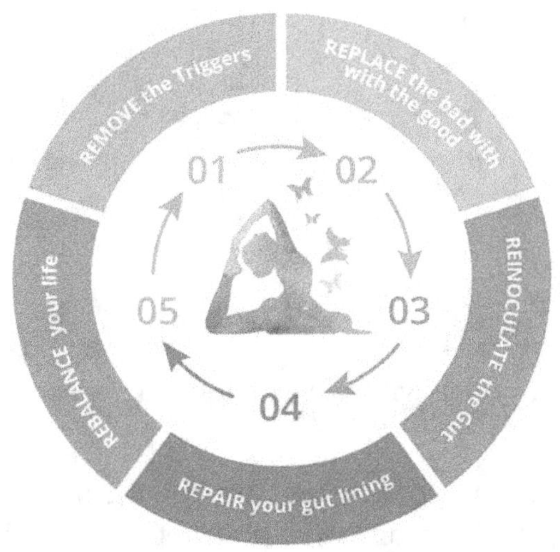

Time to add some more good stuff to your gut

Reinoculate refers to introducing pre- and probiotic foods to your diet.

Many things can imbalance your gut's microbiome. Antibiotics and ageing are two common ways the gut microbiome can change. When there is an imbalance of bacteria, your gut enters a state of dysbiosis. Simply put, the different pieces don't work together as well as they should. To return to a state of symbiosis, we have to re-introduce the right kind of healthy bacteria to our system.

Prebiotics help the gut bacteria produce nutrients for your colon cells and leads to a healthier digestive system. They feed probiotics.[1]

Eat Prebiotic loaded foods:

- Artichokes
- Onions
- Garlic
- Chicory salad
- Dandelion greens
- Asparagus
- Leeks
- Berries
- Bananas
- Flax seed
- Legumes
- Tomatoes (people with ulcers should avoid tomatoes)[2]

When you go wheat free, you lose the benefit of the prebiotics in wheat. Removing wheat from your diet does outweigh the benefits thereof. One can replace the prebiotics by eating a variety of root vegetables (with the exception of potato as it is high in the glycaemic index).

Instead of jumping to buy over the counter medication or supplements, why don't you consider adding the right foods to your diet.[3] [4]

From the above, I have found that tomatoes may pose a problem for some, as well as flax seed and legumes. Listen to your body!

Probiotics are bacteria that line your digestive tract and support your body's ability to absorb nutrients and fight infection.

According to Dr Axe, the strongest evidence to date finds that probiotics benefits include:[5]

1. boosting the immune system
2. preventing and treating urinary tract infections
3. improving digestive function and battle gastrointestinal disease
4. prevent or stop antibiotic-associated diarrhoea
5. healing inflammatory bowel conditions like IBS
6. managing and preventing eczema in children
7. fighting food-born illnesses

Dr David Perlmutter in the *Regain Your Brain Docuseries* highlights the importance of prebiotic fiber which feeds the much-needed probiotics in your gut.[6] He says prebiotics are crucial in ensuring brain health as it protects the gut brain barrier. In other words, by feeding the probiotics in your gut, it prevents inflammation in your body which if not treated, will be spread to your brain.

We covered the prebiotic foods above, let's consider probiotic foods.[7]

The following are foods loaded with probiotics:

Probiotic Foods	
Kimchi	Brine cured olives
Sauerkraut	Gherkin pickles
Kombucha	Plain, unsweetened yogurt
Kefir	Raw apple cider vinegar
Raw cheese	

Kefir is great to add to smoothies or shakes. Kombucha can be bought from your local health store. Yogurt should be plain, without sugar and flavourings.

Apple cider vinegar (ACV) is made from apples, vinegar, and a bacterial culture, known as "the mother." While ACV is commonly used to eradicate symptoms from colds, flus or even acid reflux, it's also a good dietary source of probiotics.

Like the other probiotic foods, we've mentioned, ACV must be purchased **raw or unpasteurized** in order for it to still contain the beneficial bacteria.

It is crucial to eat a variety of pre- and probiotic foods, and not just one of these food groups.

Go for fermented foods

Remember that all fermented foods are a great option to support the good bacteria in your gut. Experiment with kombucha, or add kefir to your smoothies, enjoy sauerkraut, or snack on pickled vegetables.

Let's consider what those things are that destroys probiotics. Dr Axe indicates that these are[5]:

- Prescription antibiotics
- Sugar
- Tap water
- GMO foods
- Grains
- Emotional stress
- Chemicals and medications

In this instance, there are two types of people out there. One who is willing to take a pill, and the other who hates taking pills. Who are you? Do you prefer to take a pre- and probiotic combo, or would you rather eat the foods containing pre-and probiotics? You make the choice!

Sources of References in Section 14

1. https://www.healthline.com/nutrition/19-best-prebiotic-foods
2. https://healthygutexperts.com/day-1/drtom/
3. https://anufrench.com/wp-content/uploads/2017/03/prebiotic-foods.png
4. https://www.healthline.com/nutrition/19-best-prebiotic-foods
5. https://draxe.com/probiotics-benefits-foods-supplements/
6. https://regainyourbrain.awakeningfromalzheimers.com/
7. https://yurielkaim.com/foods-rich-in-probiotics/

Section 15
Repair

REPAIR YOUR TUMMY WALL

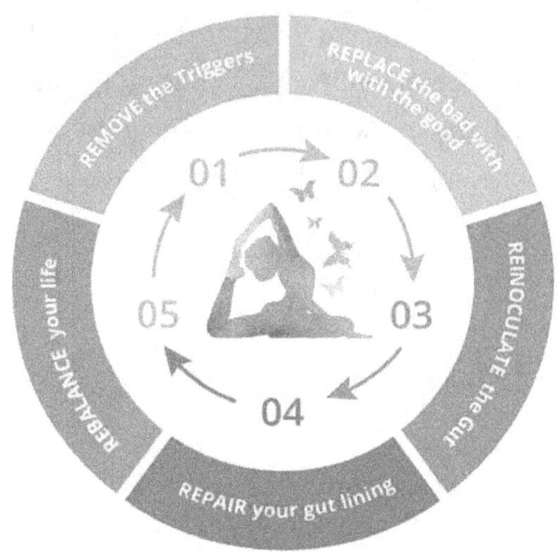

Time to heal

Repair is aimed at repairing the gut lining.

Take note that all the guidelines in this book are aimed at healing the gut. Especially removing problem foods and environmental toxins. In addition to these strategies, certain supplements can make a difference.

It is highly recommended that you work with a functional medical practitioner or an integrative health practitioner in deciding which supplements you need. It would require proper blood analysis.[1]

The following are supplements that could add value:

Probiotics with digestive enzymes[2]

Probiotics and digestive enzymes are two of the most important ingredients for healthy digestion. They contribute to a healthy microbiome. Probiotics will help to bring the gut biosis back into balance of 85% good to bad bacteria and digestive enzymes are critical to the proper breakdown of food. Also help remove toxins, bacteria, and damaged cells. Examples are Bromelain and Papain.

Remember that a prerequisite for probiotics to flourish in your gut, is prebiotics.

Consider the prebiotic foods listed in section 14.

L-Glutamine

L-Glutamine helps strengthen the gut lining.[5] It is 1 of 20 amino acids.[4] But unlike many of the other amino acids, it is unique, because it is the primary fuel used by the cells in your gut lining. Furthermore, it is helping your liver detox, supports the immune system and prevents muscle deterioration.

In this video, Dr Axe explains the benefit of L-Glutamine.[3] It is an amino acid which is a building block of protein. It not only builds muscle, it also helps with weight loss and burning fat, but is can also help heal your gut!

CAUTION – Cancer patients should not take L-Glutamine as it may feed cancer cells. Speak to your doctor!

Collagen

Collagen helps regulate stomach acid secretion, can help heal ulcers, aids in digestion and supports the repair of the gut lining. [6]

Foods containing collagen include:

- Wild salmon
- Chlorella
- Leafy greens
- Citrus
- Eggs
- Berries
- Tomatoes
- Pumpkin seeds
- Avocado
- Garlic
- Chia seeds

Collagen is an amazing healer of the gut.[7] ***The best form of collagen is through the consumption of home-made bone broth.***[8] It is made by simmering bones with water, a bit of apple cider vinegar, salt and pepper, a carrot or two and perhaps a few celery sticks. Simmer this brew for at least 24 hours. Strain and drink or use in food. This simmering causes the bones and ligaments to release healing compounds like collagen, proline, glycine and glutamine.

Colostrum

Michael Ash reported in the Clinical Education Resource that "Research shows that colostrum can restore a leaky gut lining to normal permeability levels and reduce movement of toxins and gut microbes into the bloodstream. [9]

Dr Tom O'Bryan highly recommends the consumption of colostrum, also when you come down with the flu, as it boosts your immune system.[10]

     Your Greatest Wealth is your Health

When subjected to leaky gut, you may have some nutritional deficiencies and thus your body can also benefit from a few other useful supplements.[11]

Other useful supplements:

It is best advised that before you load up on these, you get tested by your functional medicine practitioner to confirm your specific needs. These are useful for people who are suffering from autoimmune diseases.

Selenium, Zinc and Copper (Or Selenozincopper from the Compound Pharmacy)[12]

Selenium is a very effective antioxidant that defends against oxidative stress and supports the immune system. Brazil nuts are a great source of selenium.

Zinc supports the immune system and digestive system, helps reduce stress levels, improves metabolism and helps increase the rate of healing.[13]

Foods high in Zinc include lamb, pumpkin seeds, grass-fed beef, chickpeas, cacao powder, cashews, kefir/yogurt, mushroom, spinach and chicken.[14]

Copper plays a role in making red blood cells and maintaining nerve cells and the immune system. Foods rich in copper include kale, oysters, mushrooms, cashew nuts, chickpeas, prunes, avocados, goat cheese, fermented soy foods.[15]

I am sure you can see that this combination is quite potent.

Vitamin A[16]

Vitamin A is essential for building a strong immune system.

True vitamin A, known as retinol, is found in animal products like fish, shellfish, fermented cod liver oil, liver and butterfat from grass-fed cows.

Vitamin B Complex

Magdalena Wszelaki recommends a combination of crucial B vitamins to include in your daily protocol. [17]

She explains which B-Vitamins and why:

Thiamine (B1)

Thiamine is needed to produce energy. It activates Phase 1 detoxification where foreign substances are initially broken down into intermediates for excretion. Balanced levels of thiamine also allow for feelings of composure, clear-headedness, and energy.

Food sources: vegetables, whole grains, nuts, seeds, legumes, seaweed

Optimal daily dose: 25 to 50mg

Riboflavin (B2)

Deficiency in vitamin B2 inhibits the liver detox pathway that eliminates bacterial toxins. B2 is also necessary for essential fatty acid metabolism, which improves energy production in certain nerve cells. Riboflavin is involved in proper thyroid function.

Food sources: whole grains, legumes, green leafy vegetables, poultry, fish, seaweed

Optimal daily dose: 25 to 50mg

Niacin (B3)

Like B1, B3 induces Phase 1 detoxification. Niacin also helps to regulate blood sugar levels. It has an indirect effect on serotonin levels, because the body uses tryptophan (the amino acid that is the precursor to serotonin production), to produce niacin. It has an effect on the adrenal hormones.

For all these reasons, it's said to have prominent anti-depressant effects.

Food sources: liver, peanuts, sesame seeds, sunflower seeds, brown rice, whole grains, barley, almonds, seaweed.

Optimal daily dose: 25 to 50mg.

Pantothenic acid (B5)

Pantothenic acid provides foundational support for both Phase 1 and Phase 2 detoxification, and more specifically, the elimination of inflammatory substances. It plays an important role in production of adrenal hormones and is vital for coping with extreme stress. All the steroid hormones, such as estrogen and progesterone, will be produced only with ample B5 in the system.

Food sources: avocado, mushrooms, liver, soy beans, banana, collard greens, sunflower seeds, lentils, broccoli, brown rice, eggs.

Optimal daily dose: 25 to 50mg.

Pyridoxine (B6)

Sufficient levels of B6 keep the liver functioning optimally by promoting the proper flow of fat and bile to and from the liver. Magdalena says that Pyridoxine has one of the most dramatic mood-elevating effects of all the B vitamins.

It can help to correct brain metabolism dysfunctions that cause depression. It heightens serotonin production. It binds to estrogen, progesterone, and testosterone, helping to detoxify excess amounts of these steroid hormones, helping to reduce the risk of hormone-related cancers.

Food sources: spinach, walnuts, eggs, fish, poultry, beans, seaweed.

Optimal daily dose: 25 to 50mg, not to exceed 100mg/day

Cobalamin (B12)

B12 is an important factor for the activation of the liver detox pathway that detoxes the heavy metals and histamines. Cobalamin has important effects on mood and allows for a free flow of neurotransmitters. It also helps the body to secrete melatonin. She recommends B12 in a methylated form (methylcobalamin) since 70% of our population has MTHFR mutations.

Food sources: animal protein (especially liver), seafood, eggs, some cheeses, tempeh, sea vegetables, brewer's yeast, blue and green algae, chlorella, seaweed, bee pollen.

Optimal daily dose: 50 to 100mcg

Folate (B9)

Folate is a needed inducer of several of the detoxification pathways.

It breaks down homocysteine, a toxic and inflammatory agent produced by the liver if not properly converted. Folate has direct mood elevating properties and is synergistic with serotonin production.

Food sources: dark leafy greens, asparagus, bananas, cantaloupes, beans.

Optimal daily dose: 400 to 800 mcg

Iron[18]

People with autoimmune diseases tend to lack iron due to poor absorption which is as a result of leaky gut.

First point of departure should be healing the gut. Foods such as grass-fed beef, liver and spinach are high in iron, but won't be absorbed properly in the event of leaky gut.

Vitamin D[19]

Vitamin D is essential for many metabolic and immunological pathways. Vitamin D is most abundant in animal and dairy fats. Sunshine is another natural source of Vitamin D. It is worth noting that most people with autoimmune diseases have a Vitamin D deficiency.

Supplements that especially helps for inflammation are:

Omega 3[20]

Research has shown that Omega 3 can play a role in the reduction of inflammation in persons who suffer from autoimmune diseases.

They say a picture speaks a thousand words. Omega 3 fatty acids are essential for health. The website www.nftips.com did a great job in highlighting Omega 3 fatty acid foods.

Omega 3 Foods[21][22]	
Cold water salmon	Flaxseeds
Tuna	Chia seeds
Eggs	Walnuts
Cold pressed olive oil	Navy beans
Extra virgin coconut oil	Broccoli
Avocado	Spinach
Leafy greens	Cauliflower
Squash	Mixed berries
Kidney beans	

CAUTION: OMEGA 3 THINS YOUR BLOOD AND SHOULD BEST NOT BE USED WITH OTHER BLOOD THINNERS

Turmeric

Curcumin is a key chemical in turmeric. It can help reduce pain, inflammation and stiffness.[23] In my own experience, this is a wonder spice. Using it in your food or taking an extra supplement can significantly help with inflammation. Not only does it have anti-inflammatory properties, it also has antioxidant properties, and supports liver detoxification. I have seen with many people that as they start following an anti-inflammatory diet and using turmeric and Omega 3, they are slowly able to use less pain medication, and could even ultimately stop using pain medication as the inflammation in their bodies reduce.

CAUTION: TURMERIC THINS YOUR BLOOD AND SHOULD BEST NOT BE USED WITH OTHER BLOOD THINNERS

LDN

Naltrexone is in a class of drug known as an opiate antagonist. Its normal use is in treating addiction to opiate drugs such as heroin or morphine. Since 1995 it has been used to treat autoimmune disease. If you have an autoimmune disease, I would recommend you speak to your doctor about low-dose Naltrexone. It is great for reducing inflammation.

Adaptogenic herbs[24]

Adaptogenic herbs work with your body and help your body adapt, most notably, to stress. Adaptogens are a natural ally in dealing with persistent stress and fatigue because they help reduce inflammation and regulates hormones.

Adaptogens offer several other health benefits, including:[25]

- A boost for the immune system
- Support for managing a healthy weight
- Increased physical endurance and mental focus
- Reduction in discomfort caused by poor health

The most popular adaptogens are Ashwangandha, Holy Basil and Licorice Root.

People with autoimmune disease inevitably have detoxing issues. Supplements that can help the detox process are:[26]

Milk Thistle

Milk thistle is remarkable for people with thyroid and autoimmune thyroid conditions. It helps to protect the liver and supports the body in detoxification.

Glutathione[27]

Glutathione is a potent antioxidant. Its primary function is detoxification. Maintaining healthy glutathione levels prevents or dampens autoimmunity, slows down cellular aging, reduces oxidative stress, and protects you from chronic degenerative diseases. Should you have severe swelling and toxin build up, the following could help:

Dandelion root extract[28]

Dandelion is rich in calcium, vitamin C, vitamin A, iron and detoxifiers. It aids in proper flow of bile and stimulates the liver and promotes digestion. It can go a long way in helping with symptoms of swelling.

It is best to check for cross impacts with any existing medication.

Before taking any supplements, first have your doctor confirm your needs via blood tests. Please consult your homeopath, functional medicine practitioner or medical practitioner.

Quercetin[29]

Quercetin is great to help your body fight any chronic viral infection. It can also help you fight any allergies. It helps the immune system repair the damage that is done on a daily basis. It is a great general support to the immune system. Another great benefit is that it can help the liver remove toxic chemicals and compounds that could lead to cancer. It can also help in the prevention of heart disease and help prevent neurodegenerative disorders such as Alzheimer's, Dementia and Parkinson's. Natural sources are kale, broccoli, scallions, yellow onions, apples and berries.

Natural alternatives with inflammatory properties:[30]

- Ginger (delicious in food)
- Turmeric (my favourite!)
- Anti-inflammatory diet (Can't go wrong here!)
- Cinnamon (adds great taste to veggies)
- MSM (broccoli, walnuts, garlic, onion, asparagus, flax seed, eggs, kale, red bell peppers)
- Bromelain (pineapple)
- Magnesium (green leafy veggies, beans, nuts, brown rice)

It is worth it to load your diet with these.

Sources of References in Section 15

1. To find a practitioner, go to: https://www.compounding.co.za
2. https://www.hyperbiotics.com/blogs/recent-articles/enzymes-and-probiotics-partners-in-digestion
3. https://www.youtube.com/watch?v=2k3UMkXYY6U
4. https://www.smart-publications.com/articles/remove-toxins-and-boost-glutathione-and-immune-function-with-glutamine/
5. https://goodbyeleakygut.com/l-glutamine-leaky-gut/
6. https://www.furtherfood.com/collagen-protein-superfood-gut-health-heals-leaky-gut-digestive-problems/

7. http://natmedworld.com/collagen-in-a-nutshell/

8. https://blog.kettleandfire.com/foods-with-collagen/

9. https://www.clinicaleducation.org/resources/reviews/colostrum-meets-the-microbiome-a-tried-and-true-remedy-for-gut-health-takes-center-stage/

10. https://www.facebook.com/thedr.com.english/videos/1772140846150539/

11. https://www.compounding.co.za/detox-liver-support/

12. https://www.healthline.com/nutrition/selenium-benefits

13. https://www.organicfacts.net/health-benefits/minerals/health-benefits-of-zinc.html

14. https://www.medicalnewstoday.com/articles/288165.php

15. https://nutrihealthline.com/healthy-food/foods-rich-in-copper/

16. https://drwillcole.com/5-foods-i-recommend-for-people-struggling-with-autoimmune-diseases/

17. https://www.hormonesbalance.com/articles/b-vitamins-for-your-hormones/

18. https://drwillcole.com/5-foods-i-recommend-for-people-struggling-with-autoimmune-diseases/

19. https://drwillcole.com/5-foods-i-recommend-for-people-struggling-with-autoimmune-diseases/

20. http://www.rejuvenation-science.com/research-news/omega-3-fish-oil-1/n-omega-3-autoimmune-disease

21. www.nftips.com

22. http://www.nftips.com/2014/05/diet-treatments-for-breast-cancer.html

23. http://natmedworld.com/dr-bernard-brom-on-the-benefits-of-curcumin-for-inflammation/

24. https://www.drweil.com/vitamins-supplements-herbs/herbs/turmeric/

25. https://www.globalhealingcenter.com/natural-health/what-are-adaptogens/

26. http://www.naturalendocrinesolutions.com/articles/milk-thistle-thyroid-health/

27. http://undergroundwellness.com/glutathione-autoimmune-connection-part-2/

28. https://www.organicfacts.net/health-benefits/herbs-and-spices/health-benefits-of-dandelion.html

29. https://drhedberg.com/benefits-of-quercetin/

30. https://draxe.com/aspirin-side-effects/

Section 16
Rebalance

REBALANCE

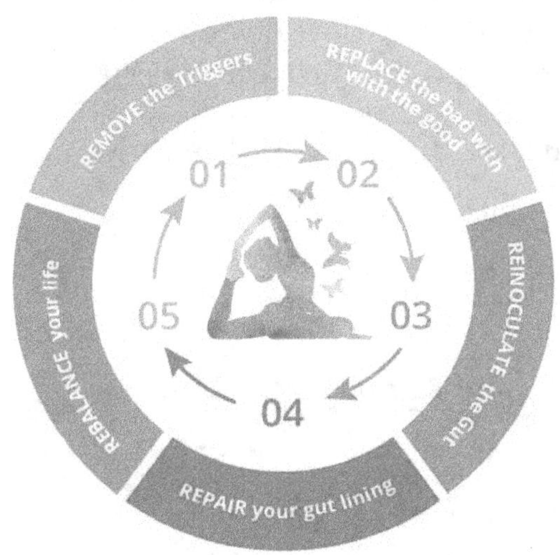

Fix your lifestyle

Rebalance means paying attention to lifestyle choices such as sleep, exercise and stress that can all affect the GI tract. These lifestyle changes also need to be tackled in a systematic way. None of us cope well with too much change. In this section you will be provided with a host of proposed lifestyle options. You need to decide what will work for you.

Make one change at time and see what the impact is. Once that change is a habit and does not require effort anymore, move to the next one.

Manage stress[1]

It starts with understanding your stressors.

What are your stressors?

We are all faced with multiple stressors every day of our lives. You might think that stressors are those things we are exposed to that could potentially have a negative impact on us. Not necessarily. People respond in different ways to stressors. Some are motivated by them, while others may experience extreme symptoms as a result. Stressors are typically divided into 6 categories:

1. Career/intellectual,

2. environmental,

3. psycho-emotional,

4. physiological,

5. relationship stressors and

6. life events.

Career/Intellectual stressors

Career or intellectual stressors refer to any work or study related stressors. In a negative context, it typically refers to stress that you are being exposed to because your career is not progressing as you anticipated, or your work environment is unsatisfactory.

We all know that in the workplace the only constant is change. Change brings about great stress. You end up not knowing where you are going with your career, when you will get promoted, what you will be doing, and so forth.

In South Africa, an added dynamic is Employment Equity. Some organisations fast track young black professionals. In some instances, some of these young professionals tend to be set up for failure. By moving too fast, their experience levels fall short, rendering them unable to deal with the delicate dynamics in the work environment. They are put under great pressure, which sometimes can have disastrous consequences for both the organisation and the person involved. What saddens me is that in many instances individuals are broken in the process. On the other side of the coin, white South Africans' careers tend to be stifled and job opportunities limited. The spirit of employment equity legislation is sound and well understood, but unfortunately often poorly implemented to the detriment of many, regardless of race.

Given the political scene in South Africa, many people opt for starting their own businesses. In the current climate, you need to be tough to cope with managing your own business. Small business owners will know exactly what I am talking about. Labour legislation and taxation requirements make it almost impossible to run a profitable business. Besides having to deal with labour issues, legislation increasingly brings about greater financial strain on small business owners. Government is introducing legislation to protect employees, but the consequences for the small business owner are not always taken into consideration. From my perspective, small business owners are the one group of people in South Africa which are exposed to the greatest levels of stress.

Our aim is to proactively manage our stress to either limit our stressors, or to make sure we are able and strong enough to cope with them. Stress cannot always be avoided, but it can be managed!

Another interesting career stressor is being overloaded or under loaded at work. I guess everyone agrees that if you are overloaded for an extended period, this will eventually lead to burn out. You will become irritable, forgetful and indecisive, which will in turn lead to sleepless nights and strained relationships. On the other hand, if you are underutilised at work, not challenged enough, you will lack motivation, be irritable, have sleeping difficulties and avoid work. The exciting part is that we all have a threshold in terms of our career where we can experience optimal stress. Yes! Optimal stress!

When you are exposed to the correct level of stress, you will feel motivated, energised, in control, alert and sometimes exhilarated. I know you know what I am talking about.

Environmental stressors

Environmental stressors refer to any exposure in your work and living environment which is potentially not conducive to your physical or emotional health. Did you know that almost everything we use in our households is toxic: from cleaning chemicals, facial creams, bath soaps, plastic containers, to pesticides, etc? In section 17 we will review environmental stressors at length.

Psycho-emotional stressors

Psycho-emotional stressors refer to any event or activity in our lives that is rooted in our psyche and brings about emotional discomfort. These differ from one person to the next. What creates an emotional response in one person might have no effect on the next.

Psycho-emotional stressors are mainly the result of how people think and feel about themselves, like trying to live up to some expectation and not being able to do so. You may want to look differently, have a different car, job, salary or spouse. It's all about not feeling in control of your life and not accepting yourself for who you are.

Many of us have deep rooted uncertainties and fears which haunt us for life.

Physiological Stressors

Physiological stressors refer to your general health and fitness. When your body is suffering because you are not nourishing it with healthy food, exercising it to stay fit, nor sleeping enough to allow it to recover, you will be stressed. It also includes exposing your body to harmful substances.

Relationship stressors

Relationship stressors are those stressors that relate to all the relationships we have, such as family, friends, co-workers or even ourselves. Are those relationships healthy? Or are they stress inducing?

Life events

In the course of your life, there are always events that you either plan for or not, but that inevitably create enormous amounts of stress.

Much research has been done on the relationship between major life events and the onset of illness. The impact of such events is considered cumulative. The more events you experience, the greater the impact and possibility of illness (Rabkin & Elmer, 1976). In their research they found a relationship between mounting life changes and the occurrence of sudden cardiac death, accidents, diabetes, etc. They also found that some people were severely affected by life events and others not. There are multiple factors impacting your ability to cope with life events, some of which include your personality and your ability to maintain a healthy immune system.

Death of a spouse or a close family member is one of the events that has the greatest impact on any individual.[2] Break up, divorce or marital separation also has a significant impact on a person's stress levels. In my opinion, any direct exposure to crime is as stressful, if not worse, depending on the physical and emotional scars left by the criminal incident. Another major cause of stress is emmigration (either yourself or someone close to you). Emmigration is a common phenomenon these days. It does, however, not go without great discomfort.

Once you know what your stressors are, you can now start doing something about it. All the tips in this guide will help you manage these stressors.

Keep your personality in check

I can just imagine what you are thinking right now. "How can my personality be a stressor?" I have news for you. No matter where you live in the world, personality traits can be our worst enemy as far as stressors are concerned.

The Type A and Type B personality theory had its inception in the 1950s. It describes a pattern of behaviours that was a risk factor for coronary heart disease. This theory has been widely popularised and widely criticised for its scientific shortcomings. But once you have completed this exercise, you will agree that your personality does have an impact on your stress levels. The Type A and B Personality theory places personalities on a continuum. We all know personalities are far more complex than that. But for the sake of understanding yourself, and the extent to which you place pressure on yourself and others, this exercise will suffice.

If you look at the continuum below, where will you plot yourself? Will you be to the far left, in the middle or to the far right?[3]

Type A	Type B
• Never late • Very competitive • Anticipates what others are going to say and interrupts • Always feels under pressure • Impatient • Tries to do many things at once, thinks about what to do next. Perceived as impulsive. • Fast & Forceful • Pushes self very hard • Always in a hurry • Pushes others to perform	• Not concerned with time • Not competitive • Good listener • Never feels under pressure • Patient • Tackles life one step at a time • Takes time talking and formulating ideas • Takes time doing things • Do not push self very hard • Never rushed, takes your time • Do not push others to perform

We are all somewhere on this continuum. Some of us are extreme Type A's and others are extreme Type B's. Some of us lie in the middle, which means we can move to either side as we choose. The higher your level of self-awareness, the better you can manage your personality.

If you are an extreme Type A personality, you would tend to have a sense of time urgency ("Hurry Sickness"), you will be very competitive, impatient, fast and forceful in everything you say and do. You will often feel under pressure. You will experience hostility or anger toward others not performing to your standards.

If you are an extreme Type B personality, you will take your time to do things. You will be patient, take time to talk, express your feelings and never or rarely feel under pressure. You will stay calm and collected under most circumstances.

As a type A, acknowledge that you do not have to be in control of everything!

Manage yourself

The question in your mind right now could be: where do I start to manage myself or my personality? The answer is cognitive behaviour therapy. Cognitive behaviour therapy (CBT) is a talk therapy that can help you manage your problems by changing the way you think and behave. It is most commonly used to treat anxiety and depression but can be useful for other mental and physical health problems. Let's make CBT practical.

Managing yourself is step number one on your road to sustainable high performance. Managing yourself proactively can greatly enhance the way you deal with stress. Especially if you are a Type A personality, you need to conscientiously manage your personality to reduce your negative stress levels.

The first step is to create an awareness of your emotions, your thoughts and your behaviour.

Today you need to take charge of your thoughts, your emotions and your behaviour. In the model below, you can clearly see how your emotions, thoughts and behaviour interact and influence one another on a continuous basis. If you feel angry at someone, your thoughts tend to go into a negative spiral, and if you tend to be an expressive person, your behaviour would show it. At the same time, if you feel happy about something, you will experience more happy thoughts and may even dance in delight to demonstrate your happiness through your behaviour.[4]

The theory is that if you can take charge of your thoughts, you can directly impact your emotions and your behaviour.

We tend to think that it always starts with an emotion. Reality is that the cycle could start with an emotion, a thought or behaviour. And the one influences the other.

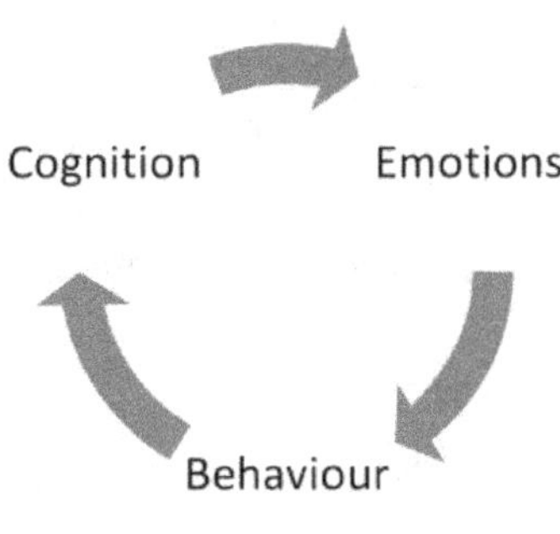

Let explore a real example. A few years ago, I woke up one morning feeling miserable. You know the feeling when everything in your life is just not going to plan. I did not feel like getting out of bed. I did not want to work on my current project. Being self-employed and having a home office did not help. It meant if I wanted to, I could just turn around, pull the pillow over my head and continue sleeping. That is exactly how I felt. But, knowing the psychology behind it, I knew that if I got up and put myself in an environment that I liked, that my emotions and my thinking would adapt accordingly. I got up (reluctantly), packed my laptop and went to the botanical gardens – my favourite get-away. I went and sat in the tea garden, not far from the waterfall. I unpacked my laptop and started working in the picturesque environment. The birds were singing, the water from the fall crashing, I could smell the flowers and the clean air, and feel the soft breeze on my skin. Within 20 minutes I felt like a different person. I was working with dedication and feeling at peace.

What happened? I woke up with a certain emotion, and started thinking (cognition) about it, which resulted in a specific behaviour. My instinctive behaviour was to stay in bed and sulk. Instead I decided to change my behaviour and go to the park, which in turn changed both my emotions and cognitive thinking. The bottom-line is when feeling bad; don't behave according to your feelings. You can take charge of your behaviour and change your emotions and thinking accordingly.

You can use the model in any direction. Let's explore another example. Are you a master of negative self-talk? If so, then you can apply these principles with great success. Positive self-talk is a very powerful tool in maintaining a healthy cognitive state, and consequently a healthy emotional and physical state.

Be conscious of your thoughts, your emotions and your behaviour and at all times be in control of them.

You will only master this principle with practice. It starts with awareness, followed by practice.

This experience is further enhanced by speaking to yourself out loud. If you hear yourself, chances are increased that you would listen and respond.

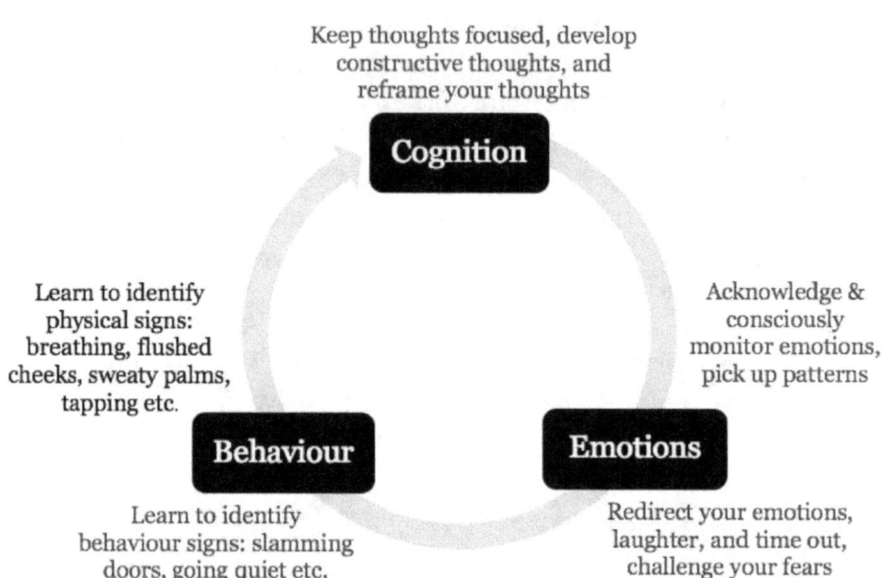

In summary, keep your thoughts focused. Always be aware of what you are thinking because it is affecting you in more ways than you realise. When you pick up on a negative or toxic thought pattern, break it. Consciously change it into constructive thoughts. Also, be aware of your emotions. Acknowledge them. Redirect them by talking to a good friend, laughing, taking time out, doing gardening, and yes, challenging your fears. You can see that changing your behaviour has a profound impact on your emotions. Just as you need to improve your awareness of your emotions and thoughts, you also need to be more aware of your behaviour and physical symptoms – your breathing, your cheeks flushing or your palms sweating.

If you pick up on it, immediately assess your thoughts and emotions, and most of all, take charge! Do something about it.

The question now remains: how do we apply these principles in managing our personalities? I am a Type A personality. I am always very aware of the fact that I want things done well and as quickly as possible (according to my standards). In asking a less experienced person to assist me with a job, I am constantly aware that I may expect the same level of delivery as I would have given. My behaviour tends to show signs of impatience. I would tap, my voice would become cold and directive, my thoughts would run off thinking: "What is she doing? Does she even know what she is doing?" You can see, in my own mind I take this 'thing' and I run with it. The more I do that, the greater my anger, frustration and dissatisfaction. By increasing my awareness of my emotions, behaviour and thoughts, I have learned to manage my reactions. I consciously change my thoughts to: "She is new and inexperienced. She has not been around the block a few times. I wonder how I can help her. Maybe I can do something to guide her to get it right." Immediately I don't get anxious anymore. I am more tolerant and don't display impatient behaviour.

It may sound easy. Trust me, it is not. It takes a lot of practice and effort from your side. You need to work at it. Sometimes you need to fake it, like I did the day I went to the botanical gardens. I did not feel like it, but I forced myself to change my behaviour. It worked! Your journey starts now...

Fight Fear

The root of all worry (stress) is fear. They say: "Don't worry, be happy". To be in that happy state, you need to resist and fight fear with all you have. In our beautiful country South Africa, we walk around with the fear of being robbed, being high jacked, our family leaving the country, keeping our jobs, and so many more. Fear is the direct opposite of faith. You need to have faith that all will be well.

You need to believe that nothing bad will happen to you. By believing, then planning, followed by action, you can destroy fear.

Let's take an example. If you fear that your family will leave the country, you are likely to be unhappy most of the time. You will feel a mixture of sadness, fear, anger and frustration. If your family member wants to leave the country, you can't prevent them from doing so. You need to plan. Do you want to go as well? If yes, then get the ball rolling. Find out which country is best suited for your family on a personal level and where work opportunities are optimal. If you want to stay, enjoy every second with your family today. Use the time you have left. Furthermore, you can explore technologies to help you communicate with your family, such as webcam. Take action to create an environment in which you will be able to maintain contact at a distance.[5]

What really helps when it comes to managing fear is to ask yourself: "What is the worst that can happen?" Let's use an example. If you fear retrenchment, the worst that can happen is that you will be retrenched. You will, however, get a severance package. At worst you will need to find another job, start your own business or take early retirement.

Through planning, followed by action on your side, you take responsibility and make sure your fears don't paralyse you.

Set healthy boundaries

By now you have clearly seen my passion for getting rid of all sorts of pollutants. Some of the major pollutants in our lives are emotional.

How many of us are entertaining emotional manipulation? Why do we do it? Well, that is simple: to keep the peace. While you are subjected to emotional manipulation or abuse, you are not at peace. Your whole being is crying out. Let me give you an example. I will use illustrative names. Jane had a long-time friend, John, that was emotionally dependent on her. He was always down in the dumps, always going through some sort of crisis. In her effort to keep him up, she pulled herself and her other relationships down. Sounds familiar?

You need to evaluate all your relationships, friends and family included, and decide whether any of them are emotional pollutants. If they are, you need to decide what measures you will put in place to minimise the effect on you. Healthy boundaries are needed.

Healthy boundaries are a necessity, not a nice to have.

People in your inner circle should have a positive impact on you. The mere fact that they are in your inner circle means that you value their opinions. If they do not build you up, but rather break you down, you may just start believing them. If any one of these individuals has a negative impact on you as a person, you need to ask yourself whether you should retain them in your inner circle. In practice, many people in our inner circles are family members. We can choose our friends, but we can't choose our family. It is always a difficult decision. But if someone is bad for you, and bringing you down, you have one of two choices. One is to remove them from inner circle, and that means maybe from your life as well, or two, you can institute healthy boundaries in that relationship. Many people battle with unhealthy family relationships. The most common example is where marriages are affected by the interference of mothers, fathers, sisters or brothers. Once you are married, the responsibility for managing that marriage lies with you and your spouse. Do not involve your families in any issues you deal with, and do not allow any interference. Place the necessary, healthy distance between you and the family members who interfere.

That may mean that you move them to the outer layer of your circle of friends. You may not spend so much time with them as before. You may not answer your phone at all times of day if he/she phones but give yourself time off. The key is a healthy boundary.

Another question when revisiting your circle of friends is: "Do I have too few or too many people in my inner circle?" If you have no people in your inner circle, you will experience a lot of stress because you do not have anybody to share your ups and downs with. The other extreme is having too many people in your inner circle. Maintaining relationships takes time and effort. Having too many people in your inner circle will put pressure on you to find the time and energy to maintain all these relationships.

It is worthwhile at this point to park a moment and think about who we put in our pavilion. We all tend to put the people in our inner circle in our pavilion. Let us use the analogy of a soccer game. If your life is the soccer game, you decided who you put in the pavilion to cheer you on or to 'boo' you off the field. That is the difference between an actual soccer game and your life. You choose!!

More often than not, we get very upset and hurt by the views of those we put in our pavilion. My best advice to you would be to remove them from your pavilion. You are giving them power over you. Only you can remove them!

Manage toxic relationships

So often we tolerate toxic relationships. If you were to be exposed to toxic gasses on a daily basis, I am sure you would have implemented some measures to protect yourself from these gasses, or to remove themfrom your environment. The same is true for toxic relationships. Take a good look at all your relationships, and if any of those are toxic, either set healthy boundaries as was highlighted above, or sometimes we have to go to extremes and accept that certain relationships only had a season. When the season is over, it is time to move on. Only you would know what is best in your situation. Setting healthy boundaries or moving on.

Accept that some relations are only good for a season

Many times in my life I have come to this realisation that not all relationships are meant to last forever. Sometimes we have a friend in our lives that is there for a season. And for that season you both need each other. But when that season passes, the relationship is not good anymore for either of you. If that is the case, let it go and cherish what it meant to you while it lasted.

Avoid negativity

The moment we switch the radio or the television on to news, we are bombarded with negative, energy draining news. It is good to be informed, but do not allow negative news to overtake your every move. Listen to the news once a day, and then rather listen to your favourite music!

Manage your romantic relationships

A romantic relationship plays one of two roles in your life. It either builds you up and makes you happy or it induces stress and makes you miserable.

You can choose what type of relationship you want to have. Be the best you can be in a relationship and make good choices that will build you up!

If your relationships and your thoughts around your relationships are toxic, you need to do something about it. Sometimes there is nothing wrong with our relationships, the problem lies with us and our toxic thoughts.

We contemplate nonsense. We create scenarios in our heads which never even happened or never will happen.

If this is what you do, stop and think about it. If you are creating silly scenarios in your head of what your partner or spouse is doing or thinking, stop it right now.

Take charge of your thoughts and instead of always looking for the negative in all situations, be thankful and appreciative.[6]

Express your appreciation towards your partner. Sometimes we should stop thinking about ourselves for a moment and start thinking about others and their needs. If we start to acknowledge and appreciate others, they will mostly return the favour. The bottom line is that we all want to feel appreciated.

I am sure you have all heard about the *5 Love Languages* by Gary Chapman. In his book he describes the five languages as (1) Words of affirmation, (2) Quality time, (3) Receiving gifts, (4) Acts of service and (5) Physical touch. This is a fantastic book that I recommend to everyone in a relationship. So often I have seen men whose love language consists of acts of service, while the wife's love language is physical touch. The sad outcome of this mismatch is that the man pledges his love by doing things for his wife, which she never appreciates, because she is expecting touch, which he is not giving her.

He starts thinking that she does not appreciate him and does not really care for him, while she thinks he lost all interest in her as her need for physical touch is not fulfilled. She feels unloved. He feels unappreciated. Can you see the irony?! They should both change their thinking and start appreciating what they do for each other.

We need to raise our awareness to the level that we can see things for what they really are. We need to avoid at all cost ruminating on silly thoughts that are not based on fact.

Finish unfinished business

Are you walking around with a load on your shoulders? Is unfinished business from the past haunting you? Is guilt weighing you down? If you want to be strong enough to deal with whatever will still come your way, *you need to let go of the unfinished business of the past*. It literally weighs you down. It wears you out to the extent that you are not able to deal with your daily stress. Let it go!

Unfinished business tends to mull around in our minds and consume our every thought. These thoughts are as toxic as they come.

I know you are probably thinking: "Easy for you to say!" It's not easy, but you have to get it off your shoulders. The best way I know of to deal with unfinished business is to take a piece of paper and write to the person/s with whom you have unfinished business. Write as though you were talking to them. Do not hold anything back. Pretend they are listening to you. If it is someone you are angry with that has hurt you in some way, tell them how you feel. Or it may be someone whom you have wronged, and you are carrying the weight of that guilt on your shoulders. Ask them to forgive you. Maybe you need to forgive yourself. Write yourself a letter!

The person you have unfinished business with could have passed away, or he/she could be alive and well. Especially when somebody has passed away, we tend to hold onto these feelings which weigh us down. You will not believe the relief it brings to write these letters. That is, until you do it.

Regardless whether they are alive or have passed on, write a letter from your heart, not holding back. When you are done, hold a little ceremony on your own where you burn these letters and see them go up in smoke. Just make sure that you do it safely. If you are not keen on a fire, tear your letter to pieces and throw it away or bury it. It's amazing what an impact such symbolic ceremonies have.

If the person is still alive and you are able to work things out with him/her in person, even better. Forgiveness will set you free. Do not wait with this exercise. Get a piece of paper and start writing this minute.

Become aware of your thoughts - – Arrest negative thoughts![7]

Dr Caroline Leaf states on her website that "75% to 95% of the illnesses that plague us today are a direct result of our thought life. What we think about affects us physically and emotionally. It's an epidemic of toxic emotions." She states that the average person has over 30,000 thoughts a day. If these thoughts go unchecked, a breeding ground for illness is created. In other words, we make ourselves sick. Dr Leaf on her website quotes research that shows that fear, all on its own, triggers more than 1,400 known physical and chemical responses and activates more than 30 different hormones. Toxic waste (generated by toxic thoughts) causes illnesses such as diabetes, cancer, asthma, skin problems and allergies, to name just a few. She urges us to consciously control our thought life and to start detoxing our brains.

Let's explore this concept for a moment. How often do you ask yourself what if this or that happened, what could have been if circumstances were different, if only you made different decisions in your life? Do you play a certain scenario over and over in your head, thinking how it could have played out differently? Are you always expecting the worst? Do you express your frustration that nothing ever works out for you? Dr Leaf uses an interesting example. She asks whether you are forming a personal identity around, for example, a disease you have. Do you speak of "my condition" or "my heart problem"? Are you overly concerned about what others think of you? Do you worry about what they may say?

Your brain is exceptionally powerful and believes these suggestions. That has a direct impact on your hormonal functions, which in turn, impacts your health. It is interesting that the Bible also refers to the power of words. Proverbs 18:21 of the New Living Translation says: "The tongue can bring death or life; those who love to talk will reap the consequences." We need to watch what we think, but even more what we say.

Dr Leaf highlights that our thoughts have an impact on our nervous, endocrine, immune, intestinal, integumentary, muscular and cardiovascular systems. In the next chapter we will look at these impacts. We will also explore how you can take charge of your thoughts and words.

Forgive

Many of us are walking around with unforgiveness in our hearts. It may be toward others, or even toward ourselves. It is like a cancer eating up your heart. Even if you do not believe it at first, say it. Say it out loud. You will start believing yourself. Forgiveness will set you free.

And most of all, forgive yourself. So often we walk around with unconscious unforgiveness towards ourselves. It is time to let it go.

Make an effort to sleep at least 8 hours a night

One of the biggest threats of our day and age is lack of sleep. Prolonged stress and associated lack of sleep should be avoided at all cost. It is recommended that you should catch up on lost sleep within at least a week to prevent long-term damage to your body. It is important to help your body get into its circadian rhythm.

If you suffer from lack of sleep, the first step is to try and identify the cause. A typical cause, but one that is many times overlooked, is drinking stimulants in the evening. I am sure we all enjoy our favourite fizzy or alcoholic drink, coffee or chocolate in the evening. The caffeine can to keep you awake. If you want to drink something in the evening, stick to rooibos or herbal tea or caffeine-free cold drinks.

A possible reason is exercise in the evening. Some people adjust well and can go to sleep after exercise. But this is not true for everyone. If you battle to fall asleep and you exercise in the evening, try exercising in the morning and see what happens.

A very common reason for lack of sleep is working too late. Most career driven people tend to take their work home. Given the nightmare traffic has become, many companies allow flexi-time. People start earlier and go home earlier. The negative effect is that most people still take their laptops home and work through their e-mails in the evening. If you work late, your brain is still very active. Therefore, once you go to bed, you are still trying to solve work problems and can't fall asleep.

If you suffer from sleeplessness and none of the above is affecting your sleep, you will need to look at addressing the root of your stress, whatever that may be in your case. Try and get to the bottom of it through elimination.

Many people that battle to sleep believe that reading a book or a magazine when going bed does the trick. Try it, it works for most people.

The bottom line is that you need rest for your body to recover. Without it your body will go into distress. A good night's rest may literally clear the mind.

Furthermore, your body cleanses itself while you sleep. The liver does a lot of its dirty work in the early morning hours. Pulling an all-nighter, or even staying up to watch a late-night show, will compromise the deeper sleep cycles that occur before midnight. Be sure to get up early as well, because you don't want to sleep through the hours when your body naturally wants to purge itself of waste. Letting your bowel movement fester or holding back your urine until later in the morning can lead to it being reabsorbed by the body.

The moral of the story is that by getting a good night's sleep, you allow your body to detox naturally.[8]

It has also been shown that chronic sleep deprivation increases gut permeability and insulin resistance.

Here are a few tips to help you sleep more and to improve your sleep quality.

1. Stop eating at least three hours before you go to sleep.

2. Avoid heavy meals in the evenings.

3. Stop indulging in electronics (television or social media on any of your electronic devices) late in the evening. We need to quiet our mind at night, so it can do its job and let us float off into sleep.

4. Disable your Wi-Fi at night. To to make it easier on you, use a timer.

5. Switch as many lights as possible off after dark. Avoid any bright light after dark.

6. When you wake up, get out and be in the daylight as soon as possible. Our brain turns on a timer and says, okay, 14 hours after this is time to sleep, and you're ready to have a good deep refreshing sleep cycle after you start that whole process.

7. Do not leave your cell phone, remote control, computer or tablet next to your bed.

In the Docuseries Regain Your Brain, Dr Breus, the Sleep Doctor, gives some helpful tips.[9]

He says one must power down at least an hour before going to bed. The first 20 minutes of the hour you can do any chores that you have to such as packing your lunch for the next day. The next 20 minutes focus on hygiene. Take a shower, brush your teeth, wash you face etc. The last 20 minutes should be focused on meditation, prayer or reading the Bible or a book that won't keep you awake. He stresses that one should have no electronic engagement in that hour, for instance Facebook, Twitter, or any other computer work.

He says if you battle to fall asleep, count backwards from 300 on 3s. He says it is so difficult you won't be able to focus on anything else. It will clear your mind and set the stage for a good night's sleep. I've tried it, it works!!!

He also suggests using a worry journal. Keep it handy, and when you start recycling worrying thoughts, write it down and let it go for the moment.

Another interesting tip he provides is to make tea using a banana peel (well rinsed). He says banana peels contain high levels of magnesium which will assist in good quality sleep.

Avoid mindless eating

I am sure you know what I am talking about. If I sit and work, and there is a packet of jelly babies next to my computer, I would all of a sudden look up and see the packet is empty. Not having been aware of it disappearing into my body! That is mindless eating. This is best avoided by not having food that you know is bad for you, next to your PC whilst working. Rather have a bowl with a few blue berries, or almonds.

Practice mindful eating[10]

Take time to eat. Sit down in a relaxed state when you eat. Take your time to eat. Chew your food at least 20-40 times before swallowing. Digestion only happens when you are in a relaxed state. Look at your food. Smell it. Feel it. Taste it. Taste the food. Enjoy the food! And ultimately, listen to what your body says about what you are eating ... your body won't lie!

Do not eat before you go to bed / Do not eat after dinner

Night-time eating can interfere with sleep, weight control and overall health. Our bodies aren't designed to eat a big meal and collapse on the couch or the bed afterwards. Sitting upright helps digest our food. It lets gravity do the work of keeping the contents of our stomach down. In people with heartburn, lying down can cause the acid in the stomach to leak out into the oesophagus, causing reflux. As the stomach takes about three hours to be emptied, waiting at least that long before lying down or sleeping is a good idea.

This touches on mindless eating. Avoid eating for the sake of eating.

Get acquainted with essential oils[11] [12] [13]

Essential oils can have a significant positive impact on one's health. Take time out to learn about the use of essential oils and introduce it to your daily routine. Remember that essential oils are highly concentrated and should not be applied undiluted to your skin. Great carrier oils include coconut oil, grapeseed oil, jojoba oil, hemp seed oil, almond oil and argan oil.

Orange essential oil is particularly good for stress. Lavender and chamomile have a calming effect. And peppermint has an invigorating effect. Tea tree oil (melaleuca) is a natural anti-bacterial, anti-fungal, reduces bad odours and can help stimulate the immune system.

Start moving and keep moving

Depending how inflamed your body is, you are likely to be in severe pain and likely to experience debilitating fatigue. Throughout this 5R programme, exercise/movement will become a key part of your recovery. But do note that given the level of inflammation in your body, it is crucial to take it slowly. At this stage it is important to not get stuck in bed but to get up in the morning, set yourself in gear and start moving your limbs. Do not fall in the trap of staying in bed. If you can only walk 20m, then walk 20m, rest an hour or two and walk another 20m. As your body starts gently detoxing, and you can increase your exercise, you can do so slowly.

Exercise has been proven to be even more effective than antidepressants.[14]

The reason is that it helps generate new brain cells, it increases the connections between brain cells, which means it aids in memory, and it aids in neuroplasticity, which means it supports the brain to heal itself.

Tai Chi, Pilates and Yoga are great options.[15] There are many YouTube videos available which can guide you. If you have not tried Tai Chi before, I recommend you try it today!

Rebounding has also become very popular. [16] Rebounding is bouncing on a mini trampoline. It boosts lymphatic drainage and the immune system and improves digestion to mention but a few of its benefits.

When I was at my worst, I found that swimming was amazing. In the beginning I could only swim one length. But the water on my skin and circulation in my body helped me recover much faster. Aside from eating healthy food, another proactive step toward detoxing your body is regular exercise.

Exercise is the most important lever at your disposal to regain your health!

In the South African context, most people think our only option is going to the gym. Running or cycling on the roads is not the safest choice. Unfortunately, most people I know do not like a gym. I have seen so many friends of mine (myself included) who wasted money on gym subscriptions by only going to the gym once or twice. Then we decided it was too much of a hassle. It takes too long to get there and even longer to get home. Let's just write it off as a bad debt.

Today I want to challenge you to think outside the box: Find out what works for you. Don't get hung up on traditional definitions of exercise. Climb the stairs at the office, take your dog for a walk in your townhouse complex or get a static cycling machine and cycle while you watch television.

When you experience stress, your body releases hormones such as cortisol, which have a negative impact on your immune system.[17] Exercise helps reduce cortisol levels and increases feel good hormones such as serotonin, endorphins, adrenalin and dopamine. Dr David Perlmutter in the *Regain Your Brain Docuseries* says that exercise is the best way to fix a brain that is degenerating. He says research has shown that as one burns calories, you grow brain cells! Is that not exciting. He recommends a minimum of 20 minutes and an average of 45 minutes to an hour exercise per day.

Exercise plays a significant role in detoxifying your body.

For one, we sweat when we exercise. The body releases toxins through sweat. Secondly, as our heart rate increases, we breathe more heavily. Breathing is another great way of releasing toxins. The correct way to breathe is to breathe in through your nose and out through your mouth. I take my dogs for a daily walk. I try and concentrate on my breathing to rid my body of as much carbon dioxide as possible. Another habit I have acquired over the years is to do breathing exercises when I wake up and before I go to sleep. I breathe in through my nose for six seconds until my lungs are full, and then exhale slowly for about eight seconds. I repeat this about ten times. This is such a small activity you can engage in, but it will have a positive impact on your health.

The best time to exercise is before meals.[18]

If you have to choose one thing to do differently going into the future, I would say exercise. Besides the physical health benefits, it also has a dramatic impact on your emotional health. It is the best way of feeling better quickly. It also has a long-term effect on your overall health if you exercise regularly.

A last note on exercise: DO NOT start too fast or stretch yourself above what your body is able to handle![19] This could have dire side effects, such as acid reflux (which could mimic itself as a heart attack), or you could release toxins too fast. Listen to your body and start slowly and build your strength and intensity over time. Remember this is a journey! ***ALWAYS LISTEN TO YOUR BODY.***

Take up dancing[20]

Dancing has amazing health benefits. It helps you stay young keep fit and be happy. These claims are actually backed by research.

Adopt a pet

Pets are amazing. They are known for their calming nature, hence the use of pets in many therapeutical set ups.

Practice hydrotherapy[21]

Hydrotherapy is varying the water temperature from warm to cold whist in the shower. It is important to never let the water be too warm of too cold. Hydrotherapy helps to detoxify the body. It also speeds up your metabolism and can help you lose weight. When exposed to cold temperatures, the flow of circulation is directed inward to the organs. Warm temperatures let circulation flow outward to the skin. Alternating temperatures unblocks stuck flows and increases the rate of detoxification and moving nutrients more readily through the body.

Get out in nature[22]

Being out in nature has an immense healing power. The University of Minnesota reports: "Being in nature, or even viewing scenes of nature, reduces anger, fear, and stress and increases pleasant feelings. Exposure to nature not only makes you feel better emotionally, it contributes to your physical wellbeing, reducing blood pressure, heart rate, muscle tension, and the production of stress hormones."

They indicate that research done in hospitals, offices, and schools has found that even a simple plant in a room can have a significant impact on stress and anxiety.

There is now better place to find God and his peace, than in nature.

Ground yourself

Grounding, also known as earthing, simply means that you walk or stand barefoot on the ground or grass.

The Heart MD Institute highlights that the Earth is an electrical planet, and you are a bioelectrical being living on an electrical planet.[23] Your body functions electrically. Your heart and nervous system are prime examples. They indicate that emerging science reveals that direct contact with the ground allows you to receive an energy infusion. This energy infusion is powerful stuff. It can restore and stabilize the bioelectrical circuitry that governs your physiology and organs, harmonize your basic biological rhythms, boost self-healing mechanisms, reduce inflammation and pain, and improve your sleep and feeling of calmness. When these things happen, you feel better in a big way. All you now need to do, is give it a try!

Try dry brushing

Dry bushing entails brushing the skin in a particular pattern with a dry brush just before a shower or a bath.[24] The skin is brushed towards the heart. Starting at the feet and hands, brushing towards the chest. Dry brushing:

- Supports the body with lymph drainage
- Exfoliates the skin
- Helps clean pores
- Helps with cellulite control
- Boosts energy

Invest in house plants and clean the air

Certain plants such as peace lily and aloe are known for the ability to help purify the air.[25] Make sure you put at least one white lily or an aloe in each room in your house.[26] There are a few others as well, check out the links.

If you have a severe volatile organic compound (VOC) problem in your house or at work, you can consider an Air Purifier.

Practice intermittent fasting

Intermittent fasting is a dietary strategy that addresses the timing of food consumption in a pattern that typically trends toward longer breaks between mealtimes allowing the gut a prolonged period to rest and recover.

Intermittent fasting can help you transform your health!

There are several different types of fasting strategies. Dr Osborne unpacks intermittent fasting.[27] He says one of the cheapest and easiest health tools you can access is fasting. Some of the benefits of intermittent fasting include:

- Regulates insulin
- Activates beneficial genes (SIRT genes) that aid in metabolic repair, reduce the risks of cancer, and turn on antioxidant systems
- Activates growth hormone
- Accelerates weight loss
- Improves energy
- Improves mood
- Aids micro-biome
- Helps repair leaky gut
- Gives the GI tract more downtime to recover

It typically consists of a 12-16-hour window of resting the gut, and an 8-12-hour window in which we can eat. You can push it up to 20 hours of fasting. This is typically done by eating an early dinner followed by a late breakfast. This ensures a 12-16-hour period where the gut is at rest. During the 8-hour window of eating, a person will consume their daily caloric need. If you can eat dinner at 18h00 and breakfast at 9h00, you can easily manage a 15 hour fast.

Anyone can benefit from intermittent fasting. Dr Osborne says the metabolic benefits have been studied and applied to numerous health conditions, including Diabetes Type 2.

The following persons should rather avoid intermittent fasting or do so under the guidance of a functional medicine practitioner:

- Pregnant women or breastfeeding moms
- Diabetics – particularly type I or insulin dependent diabetics
- Those who struggle with blood sugar regulation problems – hypo/hyperglycemics

You can still drink water or organic tea whilst being on your fast.

Naomi Whittel in the Docuseries *The Real Skinny on Fat* also unpacks the benefits of intermittent fasting.[28] She recommends one day on and one day off following a 16/8 fast. In other words, not eating for 16 hours and eating for 8 hours. She emphasises that you must break your fast with a fat and keep carbs for much later in the day. She also recommends exercise every second day, and quality sleep!

Try these simple strategies and see how the fat just drops! But more importantly, the reason the fat drops is because the inflammation in your body is reduced.

Relaxation and Self-expression

We know that relaxation is a necessity, not a luxury. [29] We all need to relax to allow our bodies some recovery time. From a physiological point of view your body needs time out. So does your mind. Your body and mind detox when you take time out.

You might wonder why I combine relaxation and self-expression in one topic. The reality is that few people relax by purely throwing themselves onto a couch and doing nothing. The best way to relax is doing something in which you express yourself. For some people it means listening to music, watching television, others sing, or you may engage in some form of art or gardening. These are merely some examples. It all boils down to finding out what works for you. Women may not like this, but many men relax by playing computer games, golf or working on their toys (bikes, cars, four wheelers). Women often tend to prefer some form of art. You have to find out what works for you and do it. Having a goal is not enough; you need to put action to your words.

I need to qualify that relaxation is not the same as avoidance. Some people throw themselves into a specific activity to avoid what they need to face in their lives. That is not relaxation. Relaxation is an activity that will help you calm down at the end of the day and give you the strength and stamina to deal with your stress in a sustainable way.

Deep breathing is always a fundamental to relaxation. Never forget to breathe!

Love yourself

In this process of recovery, it is crucial that you love yourself. Be kind to yourself. Do not be hard on yourself. More often than not, we are our own worst enemy. Not accepting ourselves, or caring for ourselves, and ultimately not loving ourselves. Making these lifestyle changes is an expression of love towards yourself. You deserve a better life. You deserve great health and energy! Every time you battle to stick to your new good habits, remind yourself that you are only doing this for yourself. For no one else. Love yourself.

Live with a sense of gratitude

Gratitude is an amazing attitude. Living with a sense of gratitude will uplift your spirit and help heal your body. Wake up thanking God for a wonderful day, for healing, for a full tummy and a roof over your head. There will always be someone who has more than we do. Rather focus on what you have and be thankful for it.

If you are at this moment too ill to walk a kilometre, be thankful that you can walk. Take life one step at a time.

Do a frequent digital detox

It makes me very sad to be in restaurants and see couples and families spending time on their cell phones, supposedly connecting on Facebook. Meanwhile they are disconnected to the here and the now. They are disconnected from their loved ones, family and friends. Develop habits such as no cell phones at dinner (at home or in restaurants). If you want to share a special moment, take a picture and put the phone away for the rest of the meal. Make an effort to connect with people on a personal level.

The sad part about Facebook and all other social media, is that it only tells part of the story. You only let the world see what you want them to. As a result, everyone seems happy and healthy, but the reality is that many people are going through rough times. Whatever it may be. Facebook tends make people like you and I that are fighting for our health, feeling that we are the odd ones out. We do not belong. Everyone else is so happy and healthy. None of that is true. Everyone has a story.

For you to become whole again, you should not disconnect from the world and only "connect" via Facebook. It is a false connection. Rather connect with people you care for and who care for you. Show them your vulnerability. Be honest about your journey. Let them help you.

The best example I can think of is when I decided to go completely gluten free. People around you do not necessarily get it. They think you are losing your mind. Sadly, you don't know how significant such a small change can be towards improvement of your health. Yet they are stuck in their paradigm. Once I started sharing some information with my family and friends, and explained to them how gluten affects me, they all came around. Now when we have family get-togethers, they would always make sure there are some gluten free snacks. In order to get there, I had to make an effort to educate them, but also to open myself up and be vulnerable.

In Section 17 we will look at the dangers of EMF and what actions you can take to reduce your exposure to EMF.

Fellowship with others

Especially if you are not feeling well, and have not been feeling well for some time, the temptation is great to isolate yourself. To disconnect from others who could judge you. They do not understand what you are going through, and you are tired of saying you are not feeling well. In actual fact, you are embarrassed about always feeling ill. I have great news for you! It is about to change! You will get your life back! But, you have to start by connecting with people. Start small. Your true friends will be there for you.

Don't judge – be tolerant

We are all naturally prone to judge. Reality is that all of us have our own story. When someone is not acting as you would or treating you the way you want them to, allow yourself not to judge. Remind yourself that each of us has our own circumstances, and we rarely share our fears and uncertainties with others.

LET GO of False guilt[30]

Let go of false guilt. We often blame ourselves for everything. If your child is nasty towards you, you think it must have been something you did. Stop taking on false guilt. Remember that each of us take responsibility for our own decisions and actions. Do not take on what is not yours. I love the mirroring technique. If someone lashes at you and they take your breath away because you have no idea what is behind their attitude and actions, it can be useful to remember that we often mirror our own issues on others. A great technique is to imagine putting up a mirror. The mirror reflects the issue back to the person it is coming from. If you do this in your mind's eye, you can avoid taking on the false guilt.

Stop fighting your circumstances

To resist your circumstances can take quite a lot of energy. When something bad happens to you, let's say your husband has been diagnosed with Alzheimer. Such an event can have a severe impact on the lives of those affected. It goes with a lot of anger, frustration and fear. Fear of what people would say. Fear of what the future holds. All these emotions can paralyse you. The best option is to accept these changes. By resisting these changes, you could deplete yourself of every bit of energy you have. I know this is not easy. Hang in there.

Meditate

Meditation has various benefits. It reduces stress, improves concentration, it benefits immune health and slows aging.[31]

Meditation does not have to be complicated. It merely means you take time out and become still. Start focusing on your breath.[32] [33]

Feel where your breath comes in your nostrils, and where it is when you exhale. Imagine your breath going in as you inhale, and your breath going out as you exhale. Try to focus on your breath. You will notice that your attention strays, some thoughts or feelings or sounds drag you away from focusing on your breathing. Don't worry when you notice your mind drifting all over the place. Everyone does that, that's how our minds are in our ordinary lives.[34] When you notice your mind has been dragged away from focusing on your breath, don't get worried, just bring your focus back to your breath. Don't make any effort to avoid having thoughts and feelings. That's how our minds function, we have endless thoughts. The idea is to notice these thoughts that have dragged you away from your focus (mindfulness in other words), and then to bring your attention back to your breathing.

Take time out and try and meditate at least once a day for a few minutes. Choose a quiet spot where you will not be disturbed.

Build in recovery time[35]

Recovery time is an interesting concept. It is closely related to relaxation. For the body to keep up with its challenges, it needs continual breaks that will allow it some recovery time. If you are studying, take a ten-minute break every two hours. You will note the difference in your ability to maintain the pace. If you work in an office, do the same. Take a walk outside and get some sun therapy (free Vitamin D injection). Just taking a few minutes' 'time out' makes all the difference.

Do not use over the counter drugs unless really needed[36]

Dr. David Perlmutter to *Regain Your Brain* highlights that the use of acid blockers is extremely common and increases your risk of Alzheimers. Proper stomach acid production is vital to unlocking perfect digestion.[37] More often than not it is thought that we have too much acid and then we revert to using acid blockers which have disastrous effects on our health. If our stomachs aren't sufficiently acidic, we don't digest protein properly, we don't access many of the minerals in our food, and we don't properly trigger vitally important digestive functions further down the process.

A very easy way to confirm if you have too little or too much acid is the baking soda acid test. Mix 1/4 teaspoon of baking soda in 150ml of cold water first thing in the morning before eating or drinking anything. Drink the baking soda solution. Time how long it takes you to belch (burp). Time up to five minutes. If you have not belched/ burped within five minutes, stop timing. In theory, if your stomach is producing adequate amounts of stomach acid you'll likely belch within two to three minutes. Early and repeated belching may be due to excessive stomach acid. Any belching after 3 minutes indicates a low acid level. It is best to repeat this exercise three days in a row to confirm accuracy.

Acid blockers are but one example. We bombard our bodies with pain killers and many more. The moment we have a symptom we run to the pharmacy and get something to address the symptom. It is time to take control of your health and address the root cause. Dr Osborne developed this informative summary that shows how drugs lead to nutrient deficiencies (you can find more information on his website):[38]

DRUG INDUCED NUTRITIONAL DEFICIENCIES

DR. OSBORNE
SCIENCE · FUNCTIONAL MEDICINE · COMMON SENSE · COMPASSION

Medication Type	Common Examples	Vitamins Depleted	Minerals Depleted	Antioxidants Hormones and Nutrients Depleted
BLOOD PRESSURE	**Diuretics** such as furosemide and Lasix	B1, B6, C	Magnesium, Calcium, Potassium, Zinc, Sodium.	Coenzyme Q10
	Thiazides (HCT)			
	Beta Blockers		Magnesium, Potassium, Sodium	Coenzyme Q10, Melatonin
CHOLESTEROL	**Statins** like Zocor, Lipitor, Crestor	D		Coenzyme Q10
	Fibrates	B2, B6, B12, Folate		
	Colestid, Questran	A, D, E, K, Beta Carotene, B-12, Folate	Iron	
DIABETES	Glucophage and Metformin	B-12, Folic Acid		Coenzyme Q10
PAIN ANTI-INFLAMMATORY	**NSAIDS**: Motrin, Naprosyn, Lodine, Aspirin	C, Folic Acid, B-12	Potassium, Iron, Magnesium	
	Steroids: for pain, asthma, skin conditions, etc.	A, C, D, Folic Acid	Calcium, Magnesium, Potassium, Zinc	
HEARTBURN REFLUX	Prilosec, Prevacid, Aciphex, Nexium, Protonix	B12, Beta Carotene		Protein
	Zantac, Axid, Pepcid, Tagamet, Tums, Rolaids	D, B12, Folic Acid	Calcium, Iron, Zinc	Protein
HORMONE REPLACEMENT	**Oral Contraceptives**: Premarin, Yasmin, as well as estrogen containing Menopausal	B2, B3, B6, B12, C, Folic Acid	Magnesium, Zinc	Selenium

(A big thank you to Dr Osborne who gave permission to use this graphic in the guide)

Do speak to your Functional Medicine Practitioner before you change any prescription medication

Expose yourself to water and natural light[39]

Research has shown that being exposed to water and natural light has a healing effect on the body. I firmly believe this as I have experienced it myself.

I hike in nature, which has a serious of positive effects on my body and mind, it destresses me, I get the benefit of natural light and in particular Vit D from sunlight, I get my circulation going and thus helps my body detox, I do heavy breathing whilst hiking which also helps my body detox and calm itself.

Enjoy the music[40]

Music is amazing for altering moods and subsequently supporting health.[41] By exposing yourself to music that you enjoy, you inevitably strengthen your immune system. Music therapy has demonstrated efficacy as an independent treatment for reducing depression, anxiety and chronic pain. Remember as a teenager how you loved listening to your favourite music? Go back there, put on your music, sing along and have fun.

Make use of supporting therapies

Therapies such as physio, kinesiology, NLP (neuro linguistic programming), massage, reflexology, acupuncture, chiro, colon hydrotherapy, lymph drainage, ozone saunas etc. can greatly support you in your journey to healing.

When your body is engulfed with inflammation, it is a good idea to use multiple methods to help your body get rid of the toxins, and to rebalance.[42] About a year before I was diagnosed with Graves, I went skydiving with my sister. It was excruciating painful. I never knew why at the time. My body was so inflamed, when the shoot opened and pulled me abruptly up in the air, intense pain penetrated my legs and my whole body. Only later in my journey I realised what was happening. When at my worst, I could not even go for a massage. My body was so severely toxic, that a massage would release massive amounts of toxins and my body would almost go into shock. I would be so sore and would immediately swell. If you are in that place, please work with a trained physio who can guide you through this process, without making you feel worse.

The two therapies I have found to be of great help are colon hydrotherapy and an ozone sauna.

Follow mouth and dental hygiene practices[43]

Dental health is now directly linked to overall health.[44] [45] It has been established that all root canals remain infected and become more infected over time. The American Dental Association has acknowledged this. Since much of the nerve complex has been removed, pain is not usually perceived even if the tooth is trying to tell the rest of the body that something is wrong as pathogens produce their toxins and continue to multiply. These toxins are incredibly potent, and they are released 24/7 into the draining lymphatics and venous blood from the jawbones, where they subsequently spread. Dr Boyd Haley has demonstrated the presence of potent toxins leaching directly out from the root canal tooth root. If you have had a root canal, consider having the tooth removed and the tissue around it cleaned and repaired by a holistic or biological dentist. Biological dentists understand the connection between root canal and disease in the body.

Here are great dental hygiene habits to develop:

Oil pulling[46]

Introduce oil pulling to your oral hygiene habits.[47] [48] Oil pulling is swishing coconut oil in your mouth for up to 20 minutes once a day. You must spit it out when you are done. Be wary not to spit it into your wash basin as it could clog your pipes. Dr Axe says it helps to detoxify the body. Sayer Ji is the founder of Greenmedinfo.com, a reviewer at the International Journal of Human Nutrition and Functional Medicine, Co-founder and CEO of Systome Biomed, Vice Chairman of the Board of the National Health Federation Steering Committee and

Member of the Global Non-GMO Foundation. He reports that the latest research indicates that swishing your mouth with coconut oil may be more effective and safer than chemical mouth washes. It reduces plaque formation and plaque induced gingivitis.

Dr Fife, in the Holistic Oral Health Summit (2018), said that a study has showed that oil pulling reduces the bacteria count in the mouth, reduces plaque, reduces gum disease and improves oral hygiene.[49]

Tongue scraping

Scraping the tongue, thus removing undesirable bacteria, helps in decreasing the likelihood of dental decay and oral disease.

Warm water & sea salt / Himalayan salt rinse

Saltwater rinses are good because they alkalinize the mouth and the alkalinity help kill the acid-producing bacteria which cause dental disease and tooth decay.

Rinse with Colloidal Silver

Rinsing your mouth with colloidal silver helps kill unwanted bacteria, fungi and viruses.

Flossing

Flossing is a great supplementary habit.

Brushing with natural toothpaste

Natural toothpaste is free of fluoride and a great addition to your dental health routine. Many options are available from Dis-Chem or your local pharmacy, or you can make you own at home by making a paste and mixing coconut oil, peppermint oil and baking soda.

Chew a clove

Clove has anti-inflammatory and anti-bacterial properties. If it feels like you have a tender area, chew a clove and spit it out after a few minutes.

Coffee Enema[50]

Dr Axe indicates that coffee enemas are known to flush out bacteria, heavy metals, fungus and yeast from the digestive tract, including the liver and colon. It thus helps lower inflammation and helps restore bowel function. Detoxing from metals is best done with the guidance of a functional medical expert. All the strategies in this book will help with metal detox, but additional supplements or binders may be required.

To perform a coffee enema at home, please check out guidelines provided by Dr Axe.[50]

Should you experience acute abdominal pain, do not do an enema, rather contact your doctor!

Abdominal breathing[51]

Deep breathing is an amazing tool to calm the mind and body. It is as simple as wherever you are, especially when you are in stressful situations, just start breathing as deeply and slowly as you can through your nose, allowing your lungs and belly to expand, then exhale slowly through your mouth. Practice mindfulness by concentrating on your breath going in your nostrils and exhaling through your mouth. It is good to develop the habit of doing a 3-5-minute-deep breathing before you get up in the morning whilst you are lying comfortably on your back, and the same before you go to sleep. When we are stressed, we tend to stop breathing or start extremely shallow breathing.

Deep abdominal breathing increases oxygen flow in your body and has vast health benefits.

Find your purpose, then live it!

People who have a clear purpose in their lives tend to be happier and experience less stress. They know the hardship they experience will eventually have a good result. As was said in the introduction, if you are a boat floating aimlessly at sea, you will be stressed. You will feel as though your life is meaningless. You will feel uncertain. You will fear the future. On the other hand, if you steer that boat in a direction of your choice, you will feel in control. You will experience a sense of purpose. All the anxiety of not knowing where you are going will evaporate!

Make an effort to find your purpose and set goals. Even if you don't achieve them as you planned, it still gives you a target to work towards. Life is funny; it often throws a curveball or two. You may be steering your boat to a beautiful island. On the way you will inevitably be thrown off course by a storm or two. You may even decide to change direction. The island you were planning to go to may have had too many sharks in the water. As a result, you can decide to head for another island. That is okay.

The only reason we have a plan is to be able to deviate from it. That's life. But having a plan gives us purpose and direction. Make those plans but be flexible enough to deviate from them and head in a different direction if required.

How do we find our purpose? Dr TD Jakes says that if you do not know what your purpose is, start with your passion. I found my purpose in my pain. What am I saying? Embrace the difficult journey that you have been on. Learn what you have to and share it with others. Make a difference. Don't resist. Embrace.

Live your spirituality[52]

Current and past research indicates that having a belief in a supreme being or drawing comfort and strength from prayer, meditation or positive actions can increase our sense of well-being. We may feel an increase in energy and experience a more positive outlook on our life in general. This can help elevate moods, reducing depression and allowing various immune response systems to work with greater ease and improved efficiency.

Faith starts with hope. If you have a negative outlook on life, nothing good will ever happen. But if you believe that good things are coming your way, you will draw it like a magnet.

In the Bible, Joseph went through hell and back after his brothers sold him off and he was thrown in jail. Yet, God worked this scenario to turn out for good.

Every time I feel disheartened, I think of Joseph. He never lost sight of seeking the Kingdom of God and he reaped every single benefit, eventually. Through all his trials and tribulations, God was working His plan in Joseph's favour. Joseph never strayed but kept his eye on God.

This is a decision you need to make for yourself, I just know that without God in my life directing my every move, my life would be devoid of meaning. I would not be able to cope with the trials of life. But what I do know is, with God on my side, I can conquer anything and everything!

What are your spiritual beliefs? Do you have a higher power which you can count on, where you can be safe, and who will help you carry your burdens?

Care for and respect your body

Your body is the temple of God. Take care what you put in it, what you put on it and how you treat it emotionally. If you do not care for yourself, no one else will care for you. Love yourself enough to make the positive changes that will heal your body.

Emotional Freedom Tapping (EFT)

The Emotional Freedom Tapping Technique is a stress management technique that helps people clear their minds, focus their attention on the present moment (much like meditation does), and improves their attitude in order to improve their chances of overcoming any challenges.

It involves tapping near the end points of the "energy meridians" located around the body.

Here is a link to a YouTube video where tapping is demonstrated: https://www.youtube.com/watch?v=1wG2FA4vfLQ. [53]

For more information on EFT, refer to the links below.[54] [55]

There are many more basic lifestyles changes that could work for you and could add value to your healing journey. Get to know yourself and do what works for you. These lifestyle changes must fit into your life. Hence, I can't tell you what to do, but I can guide you by providing as many tips as possible. I could have written a book on each of the topics in this section, but merely touched on each...make time to read more on the topics that interest you. It may just change your life forever.

Remember not to try and do it all at the same time. Try some strategies and adjust exactly how you go about it based on what works for you and what not. Trial and error are the way to go.

And remember what we learned about forming habits. Take one at a time and implement it for 3-6 weeks, then tackle the next one. Soon these will become second nature.

Next, we will review the maze of detoxing your environment. You are probably a bit unsure about all these environmental toxins and how to go about reducing them. Let's unpack them.

Sources of References in Section 16

1. Davida van der Walt, No More Stress, Your Guide to Proactive Stress Management, 2017
2. http://functionalforum.com/prescribing-lifestyle-medicine-2018

3. Davida van der Walt, No More Stress, Your Guide to Proactive Stress Management, 2017

4. Davida van der Walt, No More Stress, Your Guide to Proactive Stress Management, 2017

5. Davida van der Walt, No More Stress, Your Guide to Proactive Stress Management, 2017

6. Davida van der Walt, No More Stress, Your Guide to Proactive Stress Management, 2017

7. https://drleaf.com

8. http://functionalforum.com/prescribing-lifestyle-medicine-2018

9. https://regainyourbrain.awakeningfromalzheimers.com/

10. https://articles.mercola.com/sites/articles/archive/2014/03/14/chewing-food.aspx

11. https://drericz.com

12. https://draxe.com/essential-oil-uses-benefits/

13. https://draxe.com/essential-oils-guide/

14. https://regainyourbrain.awakeningfromalzheimers.com/

15. https://www.youtube.com/watch?v=cEOS2zoyQw4.

16. https://wellnessmama.com/13915/rebounding-benefits/

17. https://regainyourbrain.awakeningfromalzheimers.com/

18. http://functionalforum.com/prescribing-lifestyle-medicine-2018

19. https://draxe.com/acid-reflux-symptoms/

20. http://www.greenmedinfo.com/blog/amazing-health-benefits-dancing

21. https://healthfree.com/incurables_program_hydrotherapy.html

22. https://www.takingcharge.csh.umn.edu/enhance-your-wellbeing/environment/nature-and-us/how-does-nature-impact-our-wellbeing

23. https://heartmdinstitute.com/alternative-medicine/what-is-earthing-or-grounding/

24. https://wellnessmama.com/26717/dry-brushing-skin/

25. https://greatist.com/connect/houseplants-that-clean-air

26. https://draxe.com/best-houseplants-that-remove-pollution/

27. https://www.glutenfreesociety.org/intermittent-fasting-for-leaky-gut-rapid-healing-and-weight-loss/

28. http://therealskinnyonfat.com/optin/

29. Davida van der Walt, No More Stress, Your Guide to Proactive Stress Management, 2017

30. Davida van der Walt, No More Stress, Your Guide to Proactive Stress Management, 2017

31. https://www.psychologytoday.com/blog/our-empathic-nature/201401/how-meditate-made-easy-mindfulness-meditation

32. https://www.huffingtonpost.com/2014/09/19/meditation-benefits_n_5842870.html

33. https://draxe.com/guided-meditation/

34. https://draxe.com/yoga-nidra/

35. Davida van der Walt, No More Stress, Your Guide to Proactive Stress Management, 2017

36. https://regainyourbrain.awakeningfromalzheimers.com/

37. https://healthesolutions.com/health-e-tip-the-baking-soda-stomach-acid-test/

38. https://www.glutenfreesociety.org/drug-induced-nutritional-deficiencies-and-gluten-sensitivity/

39. https://natmedworld.com/dr-tessa-little-on-the-reflective-nature-of-water-and-light-and-its-fundamental-role-in-health/

40. https://www.psychologytoday.com/blog/brick-brick/201402/does-music-have-healing-powers

41. http://podcast.drpompa.com/episodes/2018/208-wholetones-the-healing-frequency-music-project

42. http://www.domanphysio.com/

43. https://www.naturalhealth365.com/western-medicine-root-canal-procedure-1481.html

44. https://www.naturalhealth365.com/root-canals-toxic-chemicals-bill-henderson-1337.html

45. https://www.naturalhealth365.com/root_canals/

46. http://www.greenmedinfo.com/blog/coconut-oil-pulling-superior-chemicals-oral-health

47. http://www.coconutresearchcenter.org/index.php/articles-and-videos/coconut-information/oil-pulling-for-a-brighter-smile-and-better-health/

48. https://draxe.com/oil-pulling-coconut-oil/
49. http://holisticoralhealthsummit.com/expert/bruce-fife/
50. https://draxe.com/coffee-enema/
51. https://www.health.harvard.edu/mind-and-mood/relaxation-techniques-breath-control-helps-quell-errant-stress-response
52. https://www.psychologytoday.com/blog/the-healing-factor/201211/the-healing-power-hope
53. https://www.youtube.com/watch?v=1wG2FA4vfLQ
54. https://www.emofree.com/eft-tutorial/tapping-basics/how-to-do-eft.html
55. https://draxe.com/emotional-freedom-technique-eft-tapping-therapy/

Section 17
Detox your environment

GET RID OF ENVIRONMENTAL TOXINS

Go green!

Detox your Environment

You need to take a critical look at your environment and clearly define your environmental stressors. It is known fact that environmental toxins are linked to autoimmune disease. From my experience, by reducing my environmental toxins, my health improved radically.

We can never remove all environmental stressors or toxins. They are everywhere. What we can do is manage what is in our control!

To add more stress to your life by worrying about all the stressors and toxins around you is not the answer. As I talk you through these, think about what you can change fairly easily. At the end of this section I will provide some guidance from my own experience as to how you can approach these changes.

Let me walk you through your house and make you aware of toxins you did not realise existed up to now. Let's consider a few.

Cleaning chemicals

Cleaning chemicals are a major culprit.[1] Some of the basic ingredients in dish washing liquid and washing detergent include surfactants, preservatives, fragrance, dyes and anti-bacterial ingredients (either active or inactive). They also contain phthalates (synthetic fragrance) which are hormone-disrupting chemicals. This means they negatively affect your hormones. These are toxic to the body and can cause allergic reactions, skin irritations and respiratory issues.[1]

Apart from detergents and dish washing liquid, there are toxic chemicals in a host of other household cleaning products, such as ammonia, toilet cleaners, bathroom cleaners, window cleaners, bleach and so forth.

I will refrain from going into detail of what each of these chemicals is capable of. If you wish to learn more, look at the links provided at the end of this section.

I would like to help you make better decisions when buying cleaning chemicals. You should look for the following:

- Plant-based surfactants (or just plain soap)
- Dye-free
- 1,4 Dioxane-free
- Phthalate-free
- Petrochemical-free
- Glycol-free
- Phosphate-free
- Caustic-free

There are many organic, toxin-free alternatives on the market. Or even easier, you can make your own.

A simple recipe for a general household cleaner is:
1. A cup of white vinegar
2. A cup of water
3. 3-5 drops lemon essential oil
4. 3-5 drops tea tree essential oil

Mix in a spray bottle, and use in the kitchen, or in the bathroom. You can even use this solution to clean tiles.

Alternatively, there are so many great stores and online stores where one can get non-toxic alternatives. My favourites are

- Faithful to Nature https://www.faithful-to-nature.co.za/
- Jacksons Real Food Market http://jacksonsrealfoodmarket.co.za
- Wellness Warehouse https://www.wellnesswarehouse.com/

Should you buy essential oils, or green products, take care to read labels. Many products are sold as natural, but still contains preservatives, fragrances and parabens which are endocrine disrupters. Essential oils must be 100% pure, and green products should not contain any chemical compounds.

In South Africa we have many options, Pick n Pay, as well as Woolworths, Builder's Warehouse and Dis-Chem have green ranges.

Indoor air contamination[2]

Indoor air contamination comes from various sources, such as toxins trapped in carpets, flame retardant treatments in your upholstery and paint on walls.[3] Volatile organic compounds (VOCs), which are airborne chemicals implicated in a range of ill health effects, should be limited in your home.[4] Ideally speaking we should replace our sofas and mattresses with products that are made from flame retardant material with non-toxic options.

The best option for a mattress is an organic latex mattress, without any flame retardants or polyurethane.

Changing our bedding and furniture is likely to be a challenge for most of us. If you can, replace all composite wood that go by names such as pressed wood, compressed wood, plywood, particle board, or medium density fibreboard (MDF). These all omit VOCs. Replace furniture with 100% solid wood if possible.

Unfortunately, wood needs furniture polish, which can be even more toxic. Furniture polish contains hydrocarbons (waxes, oils, organic solvents), which can cause a whole range of symptoms. **A product that I have grown to love is coconut oil.** It is a fantastic alternative to furniture polish. You can use very little and will be surprised how much it nourishes your wooden furniture.

You can also invest in a good quality vacuum cleaner (a HEPA-sealed model), which ensures that dust and toxins stay sealed inside the filter. It is better to vacuum and wet mop than to sweep.

Another option is to get rid of your carpets and replace them with tiles.

And finally, if you can, repaint your home with non-toxic paints. Visit your local paint dealer and enquire about eco paints.

As was mentioned before, get some air purifying plants for your home.

BPA

Bisphenol A, also known as BPA, is an industrial chemical that is used in the manufacture of certain plastics and resins. It is used in containers that store food and beverages. It is also used to coat the inside of metal products, such as food cans, bottle tops, plastic containers and water supply lines.

Exposure to BPA is a concern because of its possible health effects on the brain, behaviour and prostate glands of foetuses, infants and children.

Steps you can take to reduce your exposure are:

1. Use BPA-free products – a good idea is to replace all plastic containers with glass ones.

2. Use alternatives, such as glass, porcelain or stainless-steel containers for hot foods and liquids, instead of plastic containers. A cost-effective measure is to buy glass jam jars and use them to store food.

3. Reduce your use of canned foods since most cans are lined with BPA-containing resin, and can lead to metal toxicity.

1. Avoid heating any plastic containers. The same goes for leaving plastic water bottles in cars that are exposed to the sun. Rather use a glass bottle.

2. If you buy a take away coffee, do not use the plastic lid. Or get yourself a stainless-steel coffee cup that will also keep your coffee warm. Take it with to your favourite coffee shop.

Tap water

Dr Edward Group (2016) published a very enlightening article on the 12 toxins in tap water. Most of these toxins cannot even be pronounced. I would like to discuss four of these: fluoride, chlorine, lead and mercury. If you are interested in the rest, refer to the link below. [5]

Fluoride is a neurotoxin and an endocrine disruptor. It can harm the thyroid gland and calcify the pineal gland. Chlorine is a reactive chemical that bonds with water, including the water in your gut, to produce poisonous hydrochloric acid. Chlorine exposure can cause respiratory issues and damage cells. Lead is toxic to almost every organ in your body. Mercury is extremely toxic and can cause multiple illnesses.

I am sure you must be thinking that this cannot be true and that the amounts must be so low that it will not have an effect. Something I have realised over the last few years is that the compounding effect of the multiple toxins we are exposed to can severely affect our health. It is not so much that we are using one product loaded with chemicals. Reality is that we use hundreds. Our bodies simply get to a point where they can't handle it anymore.

I have taken multiple measures to reduce the toxin load I am exposed to. Believe me, I am reaping the benefits!

Boiling water certainly helps as it kills bacteria. Unfortunately, it does not remove toxins like fluoride. **The best solution is to change to filtered water.** Filtering clears out many safety concerns like bacteria, heavy metals and pesticides. You can either buy your water from a recognised water supplier or fit your kitchen with a high-quality water filter. Do note that some water filters do not remove fluoride.

Remember to also cook your food in filtered water.

Caution: Most water filters also remove all the minerals from the water. It is crucial to drink water that has been re-mineralised.

Beauty products

This is a very sensitive subject. When I started removing toxins from my immediate environment, I soon learned that my perfume had the worst effect on my health. The moment I stopped using my perfume, my health improved. Many of you will resist this step with everything in you. I can relate...but please believe me that you are poisoning yourself. If you have an autoimmune disease, try and not use your standard perfume for one week and see what happens!

Perfume contains phthalates and fragrances which are endocrine disrupters. To protect trade secrets, perfume manufacturers are allowed to withhold fragrance ingredients. Consumers can't rely on labels to know what hazards may lurk inside that bottle of perfume.

Fortunately, we have some healthy alternatives available at leading pharmacies and health shops. I prefer making my own using essential oils. I had severe chemical sensitivities. I used to be so sensitive to perfumes that if I sat in church next to someone wearing heavy perfume, my head started to pound, I would itch all over and my eyes would swell. I would go so far to say that changing my perfume and cleaning chemicals to natural alternatives had the biggest positive impact on my health. Over and above the removal of gluten from my diet. Today my chemical sensitivity has reduced almost 100%. Occasionally a severe exposure will make my body react.

Just as perfume is loaded with toxic fragrances which manufacturers do not have to divulge, so are bath soaps and creams, sunscreen, shampoos, facial creams and so forth. I replaced all my facial products with rooibos extract and aloe-based products which have no toxic ingredients.

If you buy fragrance free, non-toxic creams, you can simply add a few drops of essential oils. **The typical rule is 2-3 drops for every 10ml of oil or cream.** Coconut oil is a great option. For perfume, I mix a few drops surgical alcohol with distilled water, and simply add a nice mix of essential oils. Great options are Frankincense, Ylang Ylang, Lilac and Tea Tree Oil. You need to play around and find a mix that works for you.

Just a few notes on essential oils.[7] According to Dr Axe, the following essential oils should not be used during pregnancy:

Basil	Cinnamon	Eucalyptus	Manuka
Birch	Citronella	Fennel	Marjoram
Black pepper	Clary sage	Geranium (not considered safe during first trimester)	Melissa
Cedarwood	Clove	Hyssop	Myrrh
Cardamom	Cumin	Jasmine	Oregano
Cassia	Cypress	Lemongrass	Tea Tree

If you have cats, make sure to avoid them getting in contact with basil, birch, cinnamon, clove, fennel, melaleuca, nutmeg, oregano, peppermint, thyme, rosemary, spearmint, and wintergreen, bergamot, dill, grapefruit, lemon, lime, orange, and tangerine.[8]

And dogs should not have contact with Melaleuca (Tea Tree), Birch, Camphor, and Wintergreen.

Another unsuspected culprit is cosmetics. An excellent website to visit is: www.safecosmetics.org.

This website started a campaign for safe cosmetics.[9] They discuss all the cosmetic ingredients that should raise your eyebrows. They highlight toxic ingredients in products such as sunscreen, make-up, creams, shampoos and conditioners, hairspray, personal care products, soaps, detergents, toothpastes and deodorants, to mention but a few. It is worth it to invest in toxic free, green cosmetic products. To my surprise these healthy, non-toxic alternatives are fairly priced.

I personally use Bionike and find it to be very effective. In South Africa, it is available from Dis-Chem.

It is important to note that cosmetics may also contain gluten. This is what you have to look out for:

- Glutens[10]
- Flours
- Extracts such as barley extract, or fermented grains, hydrolysed malt extract, vulgare (wheat) germ oil, yeast extract
- Proteins such as hydrolysed vegetable protein and hydrolysed wheat protein
- Starches such as hydrolysed wheat starch
- Dextrins: Dextrin and maltodextrin

If you are sensitive to gluten, or you suspect you are sensitive to gluten, you should please make an effort to eliminate all gluten from your diet and personal care product exposure.[11]

Getting back to natural alternatives. Dr Axe wrote an article where he outlines 77 uses of coconut oil.[12] Take the time to check out the link provided.

I regularly use coconut oil for the following:

1. Furniture polish
2. Body lotion
3. Hair mask/conditioner
4. Homemade toothpaste, mixed with bicarbonate of soda to form a paste
5. Natural deodorant – mix a little bicarbonate of soda and essential oils – it is amazing, especially when you exercise. It completely neutralises the smell of sweat. Or add some non-toxic cream or shea butter, and add a few drops of essential oil.
6. Sunscreen[13] – SPF is a measure of how much UV radiation is blocked. Coconut Oil has an SPF of 4, which blocks 75% of UV radiation. 75% protection is about 45 minutes of sun exposure. An SPF 15 blocks 94%, an SPF 30 blocks 97%, and SPF of 40 blocks 98%. Anything above this only offers minimal additional protection.
7. Insect repellent: mix a tablespoon of coconut oil with a couple of drops of peppermint, rosemary, and tea tree oil to repel flies and mosquitoes.[14] Adding cintronella essntial oil also works wonders.

Seeing that I mentioned toothpaste in the list above, it is worthwhile to mention that it is loaded with fluoride which interferes with your thyroid function. Dr Robert Scott Bell, in the Holistic Oral Health

Summit (2018), says it also leads to greater uptake of metals by the body, thus leading to metal toxicity. Can you believe it!! Shocking! Anyway, Dis-Chem has a great range of natural toothpaste options.

You can literally get all your personal care needs by ordering online from:

1. Faithful to Nature https://www.faithful-to-nature.co.za/
2. Or Wellness Warehouse https://www.wellnesswarehouse.com/

When you go to your local pharmacy or health shop, take care to read labels. Many products are sold as natural, but still contain preservatives, fragrances and parabens which are endocrine disrupters.

To date I have replaced all my facial products, body creams, shower gels, hair products, make-up, deodorants and perfumes with natural products. I used to buy quite a few but have taken the time to learn how to make some myself. The impact on my health has been incredible. If you battle with constant allergies, chemical sensitivities or asthma, I highly recommend that you try detoxing your environment.

Laundry detergents

Earlier I mentioned the toxicity in laundry detergents and fabric softeners. They also contain hormone disrupting fragrances. A great alternative is bicarbonate of soda, better known as baking soda. You will be surprised; you won't even need softener.

If you are not sure where to start with detoxing your environment, this could be a simple change you make that could have a major impact on your health.

You are exposed 24/7 to your clothes and bedding.[15] By removing this toxic load, you will feel better within a day. Get rid of your washing detergent and give bicarbonate of soda (baking soda) a try. Use exactly the same amount as you would for laundry detergent. If your washing has a bad odour, such as your dog blankets, you can add a bit of white vinegar. It will remove all smells. If you are looking for a fresh smell, just add a few drops essential oil.

If you wish to consider other options, check out natural ranges from your local health shop, or consider a variety of options from Faithful to Nature.[15]

Air fresheners

Air fresheners are loaded with VOCs that are highly toxic. They also contain phthalates which were mentioned earlier. These are hormone-disrupting chemicals. Sarah Corriher published a very interesting article on this subject. [16]

There are multiple non-toxic alternatives on the market which use a blend of essential oils. They smell fresh and do not harm your body. Do yourself a favour and visit your local health shop. Or make your own by mixing distilled water, a few drops of alcohol and your choice of essential oils. Remember the golden rule, 2-3 drops per 10ml.

Insecticides and pesticides

We all know that household insecticides and pesticides should be toxic. They are designed to get rid of pests. Unfortunately, they are just as toxic to humans.

Derek Markham (2016) shares some very interesting homemade insecticide recipes. [17] There are products on the market which are bio-degradable and less toxic. They are more expensive, but effective. And most importantly, they do not lead to respiratory illnesses.

Have you ever wondered why some cultures leave their shoes at the door? If you walk around stepping into pesticides, and you go home, you spread it in your home. Especial if you have small children in your home, it's highly recommended to adopt this habit. If baby crawls on the floor, he or she gets directly affected by pesticides.

It was mentioned earlier that most of the foods we are exposed to are just as toxic as a result of pesticides.[18] A friendly reminder to rather go for organic foods.

A great product for general use in your house is Biokill. It is available at PnP Hyper Markets and Builder's Warehouse.

Exhaust fumes

Exposure to exhaust fumes is inevitable. Most of us are stuck in traffic on a daily basis. I have developed the habit of closing my air vents when in dense traffic. It at least helps to keep some of the toxins out. Another strategy is to change your route to work to one that carries less traffic. Or if you can, work flexi-hours and avoid heavy traffic all together.

Fire place smoke

We all love a fireplace. It creates a cosy and warm atmosphere. The Cleveland Clinic published an article on their website to highlight the dangers of fireplace smoke. [19]

The best solution is to limit your exposure by installing a fireplace with a door which closes tightly and doesn't emit smoke into the house.

Non-stick pots and pans

I am sure you love your non-stick pans. Unfortunately, they are covered with a synthetic polymer which is toxic. The Environmental Working Group (EWG) unpacks the dangers of using non-stick pans.[20] They indicate that when heated, it releases toxic fumes that may kill pet birds and cause people to develop flu-like symptoms. Aluminium cookware can also leach aluminium.

This is another easy change to make.

Safer options are stainless steel, ceramic or cast-iron pots and pans. One way to limit your risk with a non-stick pan is to cook your food over low temperatures. The best option though, is get rid of your non-stick pots and pans.

It took me 3 years to make all the changes listed in this book. Take it one day at a time and do what you can within your budget.

Ergonomics

Ergonomics refer to the way your physical environment is set up. You are now probably wondering what that has to do with stress management.

To practice a proactive stress management philosophy, you need to make sure that your physical living and work environment is set up to produce the least amount of stress to your body.

Consideration should be given to the lighting where you live and work, the height of your office chair, the positioning of your phone and the direction of your computer screen relative to the window in your office. As for the height of your seat, it is optimal once your elbows are at a 90-degree angle with the desk. That way you remove pressure from your neck. If you suffer from chronic neck stiffness, your first step should be to review the height of your seat relative to your desk.

If you are left-handed, it is best to position your phone on the right-hand side of your computer and the opposite if you are right-handed.

Another potentially major stressor to your body is the way your seat is positioned in your car, your office and in front of the television. You should always sit as upright as possible with support to your lower back. A few years ago I suffered from chronic back ache. I tried everything to get rid of it. I then looked for the root cause of my back ache. I always try to identify the cause, so that I can address the problem at its root and not treat the symptoms. I analysed when my back ache started. I soon realised it started just when I bought my new car. What a light bulb moment! Yes, my new car seat wasn't positioned correctly. I travel a lot, and the seat positioning put so much strain on my back that I could barely handle it. Once I found the correct position of the seat, I still had to do a bit of physiotherapy to get rid of the spasm, but the chronic backache was something of the past. If you spend a lot of time in your car, ensure your seat is positioned such that it supports your back, rather than putting strain on it.

Most living room chairs don't provide proper support to the lower back, which can lead to chronic lower back ache. If you suffer from lower back pain, take a look at the chairs you use and determine whether it gives you the support you need.

One last example I need to mention is the exercise equipment you use. Due to crime levels in South Africa, we tend to try and spend some time in the gym, or even set up home gyms. Gym equipment is designed such that you can adapt it to the length or build of the person using the equipment. I have found that when I do go to the gym, I am often too lazy to adjust the equipment to my height. Inevitably it then puts strain on me rather than doing any good. Rather adjust the equipment to fit your body, otherwise your effort to manage your stress via exercise becomes one of your stressors.

These are a few examples just to make you aware of the impact of poor or good ergonomics on your body.

Clean out your shower head

Nontuberculous Mycobacteria is bacteria that occurs naturally in water and soil but has also found its way into plenty of showerheads.[21] These can cause pneumonia. If you have a plastic shower head, rather replace it with a steel one, and wash it once in a while by soaking it in vinegar for an hour and then cleaning it with a brush.

Keep your home mould free

Mould can be disastrous to your health. Mould is highly toxic.[22] Mould can create a collection of symptoms such as fatigue, cognitive issues, allergies, unexpected weight gain, depression, joint and muscle pain and other neurological problems. Many people who suffer from mould exposure, are misdiagnosed. They are typically treated for depression. What is interesting is that some people are super sensitive to mould and others are not. This is due to genetic predisposition.

If you have mould exposure, it is best to speak to a functional health practitioner.[23]

It is also recommended that you should not eat mouldy foods. It is interesting that wheat and nuts can be mouldy without us seeing with the visible eye. Anti-fungal foods can help, which include broccoli, garlic, coconut oil, ginger, celery, avocado and chicken. If you think you have an issue with mouldy foods, change your diet and see what happens.

Electronic equipment and EMF

Electronic devices are a complex mixture of several hundred components. A mobile phone, for example, contains 500 to 1000 components. Many of these contain toxic heavy metals such as lead, mercury, cadmium and beryllium, as well as hazardous chemicals, such as brominated flame retardants. Polluting polyvinyl chloride (PVC) plastic is also frequently used.

Two commonly used items that affect us without us necessarily knowing it are cell phones and television remote controls. The electromagnetic radiation is harmful.

David Morehouse unpacks research on the topic and provides some tips on how to reduce your exposure. [24]

He suggests the following:

- Use a high-quality headset and use it all the time. Avoid holding a phone up to your head. Or alternatively use the speaker phone and keep the phone away from your head.
- The lower your battery level on the phone, the harder the phone works to interrogate the microwave towers it communicates with. This results in more electromagnetic radiation being produced. Therefore, it is best to keep your phone charged and rather use a landline when your cell phone battery is low.
- Signal strength is also a factor. If the signal strength is low, your cell phone must pump out more radiation, again increasing its detrimental effect. Try not to use the phone unless the signal strength is near 100% or use a landline.
- If you carry your phone in your pants pocket, purchase a shielding device that will keep it from radiating your private parts.
- Avoid using your cell phone in a car as the shielding and tinting on newer automobiles cause the electromagnetic waves to bounce back and forth inside the vehicle, exposing you and your passengers to increased levels of radiation.
- Limit your child's use of a cell phone and do not put your router in your child's bedroom!

Dr Alan Christianson did a test for himself, using an EMF meter and checking all equipment in his home.[25] His major conclusions were that you need to be at least 1-2 feet from an object to reduce your exposure. Surprisingly he found that his hair dryer had the worst electromagnetic waves. He also warns that carrying a cell phone in a shirt or pants' pocket could provide unwanted exposure.

When you go to bed, to protect yourself, make sure <u>not</u> to leave your cell phone, remote control, computer or tablet next to your bed or even under your pillow (which means next to your head!).

And switch you WiFi off when you go to bed. The best option is to put your WiFi on a timer. Or even better, wire your house or office such that you can switch off the WiFi and rather use a wired connection.

EMF exposure should be taken seriously. It has been ignored for a very long time, and many activists are now making people aware of the dangers if EMF. Three resources that are worthwhile include:

1. Devra Davies - https://ehtrust.org/about/dr-devra-davis/

   If you got to YouTube and type in Devra Davies, you will find multiple videos that will blow your mind! She indicates how tumours are related to cell phone use.

2. Loyd Burrel - https://www.electricsense.com/

   Loyd is leading awareness campaigns relating to EMF. Take the time to check him out.

3. Nick Peneault - https://theemfguy.com/

   Nick calls himself the EMF Guy. Another great resource.

Cigarettes

At the risk of boring you, I do not want to go into all the negatives of smoking and secondary smoke. Go ahead and read the article provided. [26]

If you do not want to quit for yourself, do it for those around you.

Painkillers

One of my pet hobbies is making people aware of the toxic nature of painkillers. Prolonged use of painkillers, due to the toxins they contain, can cause headaches. Isn't it ironic! Here you are taking a pain killer for pain and yet it causes pain! Craig Stellpflug shares the risks of using painkillers and suggests natural alternatives.[27] What I found very interesting about the article is that he suggests avoiding gluten, as it causes inflammation and therefore induces pain. Just be aware that while you try to get off painkillers, you are likely to experience detox symptoms, which could result in headaches. But do know that it is worth it.

There are many natural alternatives for pain relief, such as turmeric, Ogema 3, ginger and capsaicin, which is found in cayenne pepper.

Nobody will convince me that the cumulative effect of all these toxins will not affect us. I am living proof.

I followed a step-by-step process (over years), replacing one toxin at a time with natural alternatives. It is amazing how much better I feel. I used to be fatigued and my body was aching all the time. This was due to inflammation in my muscles, because of high toxicity levels. If you are constantly tired and in pain, it is worth it to give it a try!

Please stop and listen to what I am saying: I changed one at a time.

Where would I start?

I would start with changing washing detergent and softener with baking soda (bicarb). It would have a massive impact on your health as you will not be exposed to chemical fumes in your clothes and bedding.

After washing detergent, I would tackle toilet sprays and household cleaning chemicals. Just by changing to green products such a coconut oil for furniture polish and green products for cleaning, you won't be directly affected. You just need to buy a new/different product when shopping. Floor polish had a huge impact on me. All I can tell you, it is worth it, and it was no skin off my back.

After making these changes that do not affect you directly you will notice the impact on your health, this will help you make more difficult decisions such as changing your perfume to a natural alternative, or changing your hair colour to a non-toxic alternative. The bottom line is, one step at a time! Make one change, let that be your motivator to make another.

Reality is, toxic fumes are detrimental to your health. People often get cold and flu symptoms after exposure to toxic fumes (for instance after killing a few flies), not realising that the fumes are affecting their lungs. After I emptied a can of doom on a spider, I landed in hospital for a week with pneumonia. If you want to protect your body, and be proactive in terms of ensuring long-term health, you need to be aware of what you expose yourself to. The message throughout this book is that if you do not look after yourself; your body won't be able to cope with life's daily and inevitable stressors. To reduce your toxic load, limiting your toxic environmental exposure is critical. It will help you reduce inflammation in your body.

The exciting news is that the contrary is also true. Limit the toxins you are exposed to and build a body that is strong enough to endure a lot!

In the next section we review some of the recommended foods and their health benefits.

Sources of References in Section 17

1. https://gimmethegoodstuff.org/.
2. http://www.greenmedinfo.com/blog/truth-about-toxic-mattresses
3. https://www.faithful-to-nature.co.za/home/bedding/organic-bedding
4. https://www.naturellebeds.com/beds.html
5. http://www.globalhealingcenter.com/natural-health/12-toxins-in-your-drinking-water/
6. http://h2o.co.za
7. https://draxe.com/essential-oil-safety/
8. https://drericz.com/essential-oils-for-dogs/
9. https://www.bionike.it/en
10. http://www.dummies.com/food-drink/specials diets/gluten free/avoid-gluten-in-cosmetics-and-hair-and-skincare-products/
11. https://www.verywell.com/gluten-free-makeup-brands-562443
12. https://draxe.com/coconut-oil-uses/.
13. http://chirohealthrockford.com/coconut-oil-natural-suncreen/

14. http://holisticoralhealthsummit.com/expert/robert-scott-bell/

15. https://www.faithful-to-nature.co.za/home/homecare-cleaning/laundry.

16. http://healthwyze.org/reports/184-how-air-fresheners-are-killing-you

17. http://www.treehugger.com/lawn-garden/8-natural-homemade-insecticides-save-your-garden-without-killing-earth.html.

18. http://www.biokill.com.hk/main.php

19. https://health.clevelandclinic.org/2014/12/that-cozy-fire-could-be-hazardous-to-your-health/.

20. http://www.ewg.org/research/healthy-home-tips/tip-6-skip-non-stick-avoid-dangers-teflon

21. https://www.prevention.com/health/is-there-scary-bacteria-in-your-showerhead-making-you-sick

22. http://www.toxic-mould-support-australia.org/dave-aspreys-moldy-documentary/

23. https://www.moldbacteria.com/mold/what-are-health-effects-eating-mouldy-food-feeds.html

24. http://www.bibliotecapleyades.net/scalar_tech/esp_scalartech27.htm

25. https://www.youtube.com/watch?v=lt6tvlyQsi0&feature=youtu.be&inf_contact_key=a66865f9d2c22b0d67cc1f0fdbf04a1cb3798803fb45e9aa1ad44a5ef05bd93d

26. http://www.heart.org/HEARTORG/HealthyLiving/QuitSmoking/QuittingSmoking/Smoking-Do-you-really-know-the-risks_UCM_322718_Article.jsp#.WG93oXdhodU

27. http://realhealthtalk.com/pain_I_haven't_got_time_for_the_pain reliever.html

Section 18

Food is medicine

HEALTH BENEFITS OF CERTAIN FOODS

Start the healing process

Food is an amazing healer. By now it should be evident that our diets are nutrient deficient. The biggest favour you can do yourself is to start eating more vegetables.

Remember that you may have food intolerances. In which case the elimination diet is recommended. People differ. Although all these foods are fantastic, you may have a food intolerance. For more on how to follow an elimination diet, check out the link provided.[1]

In this section I want to share with you my favourite foods, especially vegetables and their health benefits.

At this point it must also be noted that most of these foods listed are vegetables that are high in phytonutrients and thus nutrient dense. Some of us cope well with eating raw vegetable or even juicing vegetables. That could be a great idea, but again, see how your body responds. Some of us do not digest raw vegetables well.

Always listen to your body!

Avocado[2]

Avocados contain lots of fiber and are rich in vitamins and minerals, such as B-vitamins, vitamin K, potassium, copper, vitamin E and vitamin C.

Aside from healthy blood pressure, the oleic acid and dietary fiber in avocados help normalize blood sugar levels. Avocado is a high fiber food, with 8 grams of both soluble and insoluble fiber per cup of the fresh fruit. This fiber is beneficial for improving digestion, encouraging regular bowel movements and well known to help prevent constipation.

Its antioxidant properties protect the body against free radicals. The vitamin E found in avocado lowers cholesterol oxidation that can lead to heart attacks and strokes. Avocados can help reduce the inflammation. This can lower 'bad' LDL cholesterol while raising the 'good' HDL cholesterol.

Baby marrow / or any squash[3]

The impressive health benefits of squash are derived from the organic compounds, nutrients, vitamins, and minerals it contains. This list includes a huge amount of vitamin A, as well as significant amounts of vitamin C, vitamin E, vitamin B6, niacin, thiamin, pantothenic acid, and folate.

Baby marrow contains magnesium, potassium, manganese, copper, phosphorous, calcium and iron. It is also a very good source of carotenoids and other important anti-inflammatory and antioxidant compounds.

It thus supports the immune system, can prevent heart disease, improves eye health, improves blood circulation, and can help reduce gastric ulcers.

Broccoli[4]

Broccoli contains vitamin K, vitamin C, chromium and folate. It is a good source of dietary fiber, pantothenic acid, vitamin B6, vitamin E, manganese, phosphorus, choline, vitamin B1, vitamin A, potassium and copper. This popular vegetable has a wide variety of nutritional and medicinal benefits, including its ability to prevent many types of cancer, improve our digestive system, lower cholesterol, detoxify the body, and maximize vitamin and mineral uptake. Broccoli also prevents allergic reactions, boosts the immune system, protects the skin, prevents birth defects, lowers blood pressure, eliminates inflammation, and improves vision and ocular health.

Cabbage[5]

Cabbage is an abundant source of vitamin C. You will be surprised to know that it is richer in vitamin C than oranges, which are considered the "best" source of that vital nutrient. Vitamin C, as one of the best antioxidants, reduces free radicals in your body that are the fundamental causes of premature aging. It also helps in repairing the wear and tear of the body through the course of life.

Cabbage is very rich in fiber and rich in sulphur. So, it helps with digestion and to fight infections in wounds and reduces the frequency and severity of ulcers. Cabbage is known to accumulate a build-up of cadmium-binding complexes in its leaves and one of the main components of that is glutamine. Glutamine is a strong anti-inflammatory agent.

Cabbage is a rich source of beta-carotene, which can assist to prevent macular degeneration. The presence of vitamin K and anthocyanins within cabbage supports mental function and concentration. Cabbage, as well as all cruciferous vegetables, are great sources of minerals, like calcium, magnesium, and potassium. These three essential minerals are integral in the protection of bones from degradation and the onset of conditions like osteoporosis and general bone weakening.

The presence of potassium in cabbage helps prevent elevated blood pressure.

Cabbage acts as a good detoxifier too, meaning that it purifies the blood and removes toxins, primarily free radicals and uric acid which are the main causes of rheumatism, gout, arthritis, renal calculi, skin diseases, and eczema.

Cabbage, being rich in iodine, helps in proper functioning of the brain and the nervous system, along with keeping the glands of the endocrine system in proper condition.

Celery[6]

The benefits of celery begin with it being an excellent source of antioxidants and beneficial enzymes, in addition to vitamins and minerals such as vitamin K, vitamin C, potassium, folate and vitamin B6.

Celery also provides dietary fiber, especially when you eat more than one cup at a time.[7] Then it boosts digestion and weight loss. In addition, celery's high percentage of water and electrolytes can prevent dehydration, and special compounds help celery to act as a diuretic and reduce bloating. It has the ability to improve liver, skin, eye and cognitive health.

It must be noted that celery is one of the dirty dozen coined by the Environmental Work Group as one of the vegetables that absorbs pesticides from ground water. It is thus best to buy organic or to grow it in your garden where you have control over using organic potting soil and compost.

Coconut oil[8]

According to Dr Axe, research has finally uncovered the secrets to this amazing superfood: namely healthy fats called medium-chain fatty acids (MCFAs). These unique fats include:

- Caprylic acid
- Lauric acid
- Capric acid

Around 62 percent of the oils in coconut are made up of these three healthy fatty acids, and 91 percent of the fat in coconut oil is healthy saturated fat.

Unlike long-chain fatty acids found in plant-based oils, MCFAs are:

- Easier to digest
- Not readily stored as fat
- Antimicrobial and antifungal
- Smaller in size, allowing easier cell permeability for immediate energy
- Processed by the liver, which means that they're immediately converted to energy instead of being stored as fat

Dr Mark Hyman also emphasises that the fact that coconut oil contains medium chain triglycerides (MCT), it boosts metabolism, reverses insulin resistance, and improves cognitive function.[9] Coconut oil is also anti-fungal and anti-microbial, and it contains lauric acid that is great for immune function.

Below is an extract from an article by Dr Hyman.

patients, MCT becomes that little nudge to help you drop those last 10 to 15 stubborn pounds that just won't go away.

THE RESEARCH DOESN'T LIE
In one study published in the Journal of Obesity and Research in 2013, scientists at McGill University carried out a randomized control trial to compare the effects of medium-chain triglycerides (such as caprylic acid and lauric acid) and long-chain triglycerides (like olive oil) on body fat storage, energy expenditure, appetite control, and other aspects of weight loss in overweight men. Researchers put these men on different diets for 28 days. They switched the diets after a short time so that they could see differences in the same subjects. One group ate a coconut oil-rich diet, high in medium-chain triglycerides. The other group ate a diet rich in long-chain triglycerides. Researchers found the men who ate coconut oil lost more body fat, which they attributed to a greater increase in energy expenditure and fat burning. Coconut oil actually sped up their metabolism, curbing their appetite and allowing them to lose more

Medium chain triglycerides can actually help our bodies burn calories.

belly fat, as compared with the men who were on the olive oil-rich diet.

MCT OIL IS A FAT BURNING OIL
Let's compare MCTs with omega 6 fats.

OMEGO 6 FATS:
Omega 6 fats are seed, bean, or grain oils (which include corn, soy, sunflower and canola oils). Once ingested, these inflammatory oils are transported to the lymphatic system and not to the blood, which means your fat tissues absorb them.

MCTS:
MCTs, on the other hand, are directly absorbed into the blood, and boost metabolism, burn more calories and fat, and reduce fat storage, while curbing

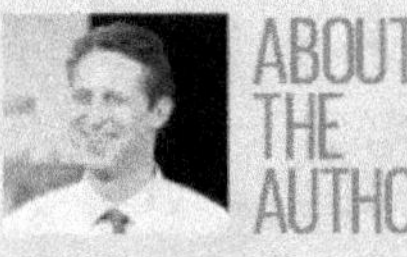

MARK HYMAN, MD is dedicated to identifying and addressing the root causes of chronic illness through a groundbreaking whole-systems medicine approach called Functional Medicine. He is a family physician, a eight-time New York Times bestselling author, and an international leader in his field. Through his private practice, education efforts, writing, research, and advocacy, he empowers others to stop managing symptoms and start treating the underlying causes of illness, thereby tackling our chronic-disease epidemic. To learn more about Dr. Hyman and Functional Medicine, visit drhyman.com

Cauliflower[10]

Cauliflower is considered one of the healthiest foods on earth- and there is good reason why.

Cauliflower is very low in calories yet high in vitamins. In fact, cauliflower contains some of almost every vitamin and mineral that you need. Cauliflower is quite high in fiber and contains Vitamin C, Vitamin K, Vitamin B6, Folate, Pantothenic acid, Potassium Manganese, Magnesium and Phosphorous. It is thus good for your overall health and a good source of antioxidants. For great recipes check out the link to the left.

Himalayan salt[11]

Pink Himalayan salt is often said to be the most beneficial as well as the cleanest salt available on this planet today. It has all kinds of nutritional and therapeutic properties, not to mention culinary uses. You can use it as a healthier option to processed salt. Pink Himalayan sea salt contains over 84 minerals and trace elements, including calcium, iron, magnesium, potassium and copper, so it does more than just make your food taste better.

Pink Himalayan salt is a much more balanced and healthy choice in comparison to common table salt. True, high-quality pink Himalayan salt is one of the purest salts you can find. It's even typically mined by hand. This is very different from table salt that involves a great deal of unnatural interference. Table salt is very heavily processed, eliminating its minerals. Commercial table salt is typically 97.5 percent to 99.9 percent sodium chloride. Meanwhile, a high-quality unrefined salt like Himalayan sea salt is only about 87 percent sodium chloride.

It must be noted, as with any salt (iodine), it should be used in moderation. A very easy change in your diet is to replace our table salt with Himalayan salt. It is delicious!

Plain Greek yogurt[12]

Yogurt is loaded with healthy nutrients. It is a rich source of calcium, and yogurt with live active cultures aids the body's absorption of calcium.

Also, yogurt contains protein that is easy to digest. Other valuable nutrients in yogurt are riboflavin, B vitamins, folic acid, lactic acid, potassium, phosphorous, iodine and zinc.

What must be noted is that Greek yogurt, still contains sugar. Make sure the brand you buy has the lowest content of sugar per serving. The sugar content in flavoured yogurts can easily go up to 30g per 100g serving, whilst the plain Greek yogurt you choose should be around 4,6g per 100g serving.

As for the fat content, it is high in saturated fat. Furthermore, it is a good source of calcium and protein, and contain probiotics. You have to look out for live culture on the label.

Consume your yogurt wisely, for instance three tablespoons in a smoothie or a shake, instead of a whole bowl in one helping.

Radish[13]

The radish is an alkaline-forming food , which is very helpful in keeping pH balance in check. The radish has detoxification properties helping to cleanse the blood of toxins and waste. Radishes contain high levels of Vitamin C. Vitamin C is an antioxidant that can help limit damage to cartilage that may be caused by free radicals found in the body. As a high-fiber food, radishes can help regulate bowel movements, eliminate constipation, which is a cause of haemorrhoids, and may help lower cholesterol by binding to low-density lipoproteins.

Spinach

It is high in amino acids, carotenoids, iodine, potassium, magnesium, iron, as well as vitamin C, vitamin A, vitamin E, vitamin B Complex and vitamin K. Spinach helps improve digestion, strengthens the cardiovascular system, nourishes the eyes, prevents oral health problems, fights skin issues, helps create red blood cells, supports cognitive function, supports bones and helps balance blood pH.

Spring Onions[14]

Spring onions are rich in vitamins including Vitamin C, Vitamin B2 and thiamine. They also contain Vitamin A and Vitamin K. In addition, these are good sources of copper, phosphorous, magnesium, potassium, chromium, manganese and fiber. Spring onions are a strong source of flavonoids such as quercetin. A health promoting organic compound allyl propyl disulphide can also be found in spring onions.

Given below are some of the outstanding health benefits of spring onions.

1. Good for cardiovascular health.
2. Help in reducing and controlling blood pressure levels.
3. Help to reduce cholesterol levels.
4. The chromium content in spring onions provides health benefits for diabetics. It controls the blood sugar levels and improves glucose tolerance.
5. Anti-bacterial properties in it help to fight against cold and flu.
6. Anti-bacterial properties also provide relief from digestive discomforts.
7. Vitamin C in this vegetable boosts the immunity.
8. Pectin (water-soluble colloidal carbohydrate) in spring onions reduces the chances of developing cancers especially colon cancer.

9. Quercetin in spring onions provides anti-inflammatory and anti-histamine benefits.

10. It is a good food for regulating metabolism and keeping macronutrients.

11. Spring onions are good against eye disease and eye problems.

12. Allicin in this vegetable is good for the skin as it protects from skin wrinkling.

Sources of References in Section 18

1. https://www.compounding.co.za/wp-content/uploads/2017/02/Comprehensive-Elimination-Diet.pdf

2. https://www.medicalnewstoday.com/articles/318620.php

3. https://www.organicfacts.net/health-benefits/vegetable/marrow.html

4. http://www.whfoods.com/genpage.php?tname=foodspice&dbid=9

5. https://www.organicfacts.net/health-benefits/vegetable/health-benefits-of-cabbage.html

6. https://draxe.com/benefits-of-celery/

7. https://www.ewg.org/foodnews/dirty_dozen_list.php#.WpkvYma B2u4

8. https://draxe.com/coconut-oil-benefits/

9. http://drhyman.com/blog/2017/06/26/coconut-oil/

10. https://www.healthline.com/nutrition/benefits-of-cauliflower

11. https://foodfacts.mercola.com/himalayan-salt.html

12. https://www.livestrong.com/article/532945-nutritional-facts-for-full-fat-greek-yogurt/

13. https://www.organicfacts.net/health-benefits/vegetable/health-benefits-of-radish.html

14. https://herbalremedies.knoji.com/12-amazing-health-benefits-of-spring-onions-and-nutritional-value-of-spring-onions-2/

Section 19
Delicious and healthy recipes

LET'S HAVE SOME FUN WITH FOOD

Make sure to get the ingredients!

Knowing human nature, we all need a bit of a crutch when we go through major changes, especially in our diet. This section will help you get through it. If you are anything like I am, I battle to follow recipes. I like making them my own. I have thus decided not to provide the typical recipes which specify all ingredients amounts in detail, but rather to let you have some fun personalizing these for your own use.

That said, I must emphasize that baking gluten free is not the same as baking with wheat flour. Unless you are an expert gluten free baker, it is best to follow the baking instructions as they come. Here follow a few simple recipe guidelines that could help you get on track.

Almond Biscuits

2 cups almond flour
2 teaspoons baking powder
½ teaspoon Himalayan salt
2 large eggs
⅓ cup butter

Method:

Mix the almond flour, baking powder and salt. Stir in the eggs and the butter. Scoop table spoons full of dough onto a lined baking sheet. Form into round cookie shapes and flatten with your fingers or a fork. Bake for about 15 minutes in a preheated oven at 180°C.

Banana Muffins

2   small bananas
½ cup coconut oil
4   eggs
2   teaspoons vanilla essence
3   tablespoons raw honey / maple syrup
½ cup coconut flour
¼ cup tapioca flour
½ teaspoon bicarbonate of soda / baking soda

Method:

Mash the bananas. Add the oil, eggs, vanilla essence and honey or syrup to the bananas and blend. Add the coconut oil, tapioca flour and baking soda to the mixture and blend. Scoop mixture into muffin pan. Bake for 12 minutes at 180°C. You can freeze these for later.

Black Bean Brownies

This is one of those crutches that will get you through the hard times.
1   can black beans, rinsed and drained
3   eggs
3   tablespoons olive oil or coconut oil
¼ cup cocoa powder
1   pinch salt
1   teaspoon vanilla extract
¾ cup brown sugar
1   teaspoon instant coffee
½ cup dark chocolate chips (optional)

Method:

Black beans should preferably be a packet of beans soaked overnight and cooked till soft (the next day). Grease a small baking pan, preheat at 180 degrees C. Mix all the ingredients in a food processor, except the chocolate chips, add to a greased pan. Sprinkle with chocolate chips (optional). Bake for about 30 minutes. Cut and enjoy. Make larger batches and freeze.

Bobotie

Onion
Spring onion
Coconut oil
Ginger
Garlic
Curry powder
Turmeric
Himalayan salt
Coconut milk/cream
Raisins
Egg
Mince Meat

Method:

Fry onion and spring onion in coconut oil. Add ginger and garlic to taste. Add natural curry and turmeric to taste. You can add other spices such as cumin, aniseed, clove and cumin to taste. Add Himalayan salt to taste. Add coconut milk/cream and raisins (as much as you like). Simmer until half cooked. Add one/eggs, then dish into in baking dish. Add more egg on top. Bake in the oven until ready. It can be cut in pieces and frozen for later consumption.

Bread – out of this world!

https://www.youtube.com/watch?v=h6JSrU4nf18

Cake – out of this world

https://drjockers.com/sugar-free-chocolate-cake/

Cauliflower

Steam and drain, then roast with garlic and butter on the grill!

Chai Tea

Simply add two tea bags, 1 cinnamon stick, 3 cardamom pods, one aniseed star to a pot. Let it simmer for a few minutes and enjoy!

Or simply just add a small cinnamon stick to your cup of tea. It is out of this world!

Cheese Thyme Savoury Crackers

3 tablespoons of coconut flour
2 tablespoons grass fed butter
¼ cup cheese (Tussers, cheddar or gouda)
¼ cup parmesan
dash of dried thyme leaves
1 egg

Method:

Mix all the ingredients. Let the mix rest for a few minutes. Then form 8 balls and place them on a baking sheet. Press them into flat cracker shapes, sprinkle with a little cheddar (approximately quarter cup) and top with a little thyme. Bake for 12-15 minutes until brown.

Chicken curry

Onions
Garlic
Ginger
Curry powder/paste
Turmeric powder
Chicken fillets
Coconut milk
Honey
Potatoes
Carrots
Spring onion
Peas

Method:

Fry onions. Add garlic and ginger, and curry & turmeric. Then add chicken fillets, add coconut milk and drop of honey to taste. Cook for few minutes. Add sweet potato cubes, carrots and spring onion. Once soft, add peas. Serve with brown rice with lentils and wild rice (Tastic)

Chicken livers

Chicken livers
Onion
Spring onion
Coconut oil
Spices of own choice

Method:
Prepare chicken livers by frying onion and spring onion in coconut oil. Add natural spices of your choice and coconut milk. Add natural peri-peri spice/sauce to taste. Cook over low heat until ready. Serve with sweet potato mash and cruciferous veg of choice.

Chicken / mince meatballs

Chicken / beef mince
1   egg
Coconut cream
Salt
Natural spices
Onion / spring onion
Garlic
Ginger

Method:
Mix chicken mince / beef mince with egg and coconut cream. Add salt and natural spices to taste. Fry in coconut oil. You can add onion or spring onion to the mix, as well as garlic and ginger. My personal preference is chicken meat balls.

Chicken salad

Mix lettuce, spring onion, baby tomatoes, radish, celery and chicken in a salad bowl. Fry chicken pieces in some coconut oil, lemon and ginger.
Mix olive oil, freshly chopped basil and lemon for a salad dressing.

Chicken stir fry

Fry onion in garlic and ginger using coconut oil. Add chicken strips. Use natural spice of your choice. Fry in chopped cabbage, cauliflower & broccoli. (Or use any veg mix of your choice).

Choc orange truffles

1   small orange's zest
½ orange's juice
½ cup almonds.
½ cup raisons
2   tablespoons melted coconut oil
2   tablespoons cocoa/raw cacao

Method:

Mix all the ingredients in a food processor: Spread cocoa/raw cacao on your work surface, form mixture into balls and roll into cocoa. Enjoy!

Date balls

3 tablespoons coconut oil
A cup desiccated coconut
2 cups dates (pitted, and soaked in boiling water and drained)
2 pinches of salt
Half to full cup almonds (to taste)
2/3 cup of cocoa / raw cacao (unsweetened) - optional

Method:

Mix all the ingredients in a food processor. Roll in balls, roll in some more coconut, refrigerate and enjoy!! This is a winner.

     Your Greatest Wealth is your Health   234

Egg muffins

Mix some egg and coconut milk, with salt and pepper. Pour in your muffin pan up to two thirds. Now you can play around with fillings – bacon, onion, peppers, baby marrow, spring onion ... whatever you enjoy. Just add the filling to the egg and bake until ready. Sprinkle with a bit of cheese.

Frittata

Mix egg, coconut milk, salt & pepper. Add any veg and lean meats of your choice. E.g. finely shredded spinach, finely chopped baby marrow, finely chopped peppers, tuna, shredded chicken, tomatoes, spring onion, feta, carrots finely cubed, sweet potatoes finely cubed. Pour into pan, cook in coconut oil over low heat until set. You can grate some cheese over the top. Cut in pieces.

Fritters

Fritters can be made with grated baby marrow or mashed pumpkin/butternut. Mix one egg with one cup gluten free flour, salt to taste, and coconut cream. Mix and fry in coconut oil. Top with coconut sugar and cinnamon when done.

Juices

Veggie juices are a great way to get all the nutrients you need. Mix any of your favourite juices. Great additions are carrots, ginger, lemon rind, cabbage, mint, or any of your favourite veggies.

Home-made chocolate (This is a great crutch!!!)

Mix a cup of organic coconut oil, with some organic desiccated coconut, raw cacao, a bit of honey, grounded and crushed nuts (and or seeds – not peanuts) of your choice and some dried berries (e.g. goji and cranberries). You mix in enough dry ingredients until the composition is strong enough to keep together. Drop into an ice cube tray and put in the fridge. Once set, push them out and enjoy! Keep them in the fridge as they may melt in warm temperatures. This recipe you can play with and you can add your own ingredients as long as they are healthy and organic. I find that ground nuts work well to keep the consistency right.

Lemon tarts

For the lemon curd:
3 large eggs
¼ cup (80 grams) raw honey
zest of 2 lemons (about 1 tablespoon)
pinch of salt
¼ cup (56 grams) refined coconut oil or regular unsalted butter
⅓ cup + 1 tablespoon freshly squeezed lemon juice

For the crust:
3 tablespoons refined coconut oil, softened
2 tablespoons raw honey
½ teaspoon ground cinnamon
⅜ teaspoon salt
½ cup coconut flour
1 cup almond flour

Method for lemon curd:
Make the curd. Mix together the eggs, honey, lemon zest and salt in a medium stainless-steel saucepan or pot.

Heat over medium-low heat and once everything is well-combined, add the coconut oil or butter and continue stirring. Once melted, stir in the lemon juice.

Cook the lemon curd over medium-low heat, stirring constantly, until it thickens – about 4-10 minutes. It's ready once the curd coats the back of a spoon and a clear path is left when you run your finger through it. Do not let the curd go over 170 °F. Eggs scramble around 185 °F so be careful!

Place a strainer or sift over the storage container you want to store the curd in. Strain it and then let it cool completely and chill for at least 30 minutes before filling the tart shells.

Method for tart crust:

Prepare the tart crust. Preheat the oven to 175 °C and get out a 12-cup silicone muffin pan. No need to grease it.

In a medium mixing bowl, stir together the coconut oil, honey, cinnamon and salt. Add the coconut and almond flour and stir until well combined. The dough will be crumbly but should stick together when pinched.

Divide the dough between the 12 moulds and press the dough over the bottom and only about 1/4 or 1/3 up the sides.
Bake for 8-10 minutes or until lightly browned. Remove from the oven and let sit for at least 10 minutes till it is cool and has hardened and are easy to remove. They should pop right out of the silicone cups.

Let cool completely and then place in the refrigerator for about 20-30 minutes or until firm. Fill with the cold lemon curd (4 teaspoons per cup) shortly before serving. I recommend only filling the crusts a few hours before serving to ensure that the crusts don't get soft. If you want to prepare the crusts ahead of time, don't let the crusts sit at room temperature very long before putting away in an airtight container (they get soft if you let them sit uncovered at room temperature). The lemon curd can be prepared 3 days ahead of serving and refrigerated.

Liver Pate – Home made

A great recipe from Magdalena:
https://www.hormonesbalance.com/recipes/easy-french-pate-2/

Nut biscuits

2 mashed over-ripe bananas
1 and a third cup coconut flour
¼ cup walnuts chopped
¼ cup chocolate chips (can be substituted with raisins)

Method:

Mix all the ingredients. Scoop 2 tablespoons for each biscuit and form into a ball, place on wax paper and flatten with a fork. Bake for 12-15 minutes on 180°C.

Omelette

Fry chopped onion, cauliflower, broccoli or veg of your choice. Add natural spices and garlic and ginger to taste. Mix 2 eggs with coconut milk. Once veg is fried to your liking, pour egg over the veg and cover and cook over low heat. Remove omelette and enjoy when ready. If you can stomach cheese, add some mozzarella on top.

Pesto

2   cups basil leaves
2   cloves garlic
⅓   cup pine nuts or almonds
½ cup parmesan
¼   spoon Himalayan salt
¼   spoon black pepper
½ to ¾ cup olive oil

Method:

Mix all the ingredients in a food processor. Process until fine enough, place in the fridge in a glass jar... enjoy! Delicious on gluten free toast with tomato and cheese.

Pizza

Base: grate cauliflower. Microwave for few minutes (2-3). Strain all moisture using a cloth. Add egg, salt, pepper, oregano. Mix well. Press flat into oven pan. Grill until golden brown. Add pizza toppings of your choice. Garlic, tomato, peppers, feta, high quality cold meats, cheese, olives, pineapple, mushroom etc. Grill until ready to eat. Add salt and pepper to taste.

Quick bread in a mug (Another great one!)

Option 1

Mix one egg, two tablespoons coconut flour, pinch of salt, quarter spoon baking powder, 2 tablespoon coconut cream. Add to mug. Microwave for 1 minute. Tip over, slice and enjoy.

Option 2

It works well to make a premix to simplify the process. You can double up on the mix.

1   cup mix almond flour
2   tablespoons psyllium husk
3   tablespoons flax meal –
1   teaspoon gluten free baking powder
pinch of salt

Method:

When you feel like your bread, melt 1 tablespoon butter, with a quarter cup mix, and one egg. Mix well in a broad cup and pop into the microwave for approximately 75 seconds. Pop out, slice, butter and enjoy.

Rusks

It took me many years to get this right! I played around with many rusk recipes and never got it right … but finally I adapted a recipe I found on the world wide web that tastes just like normal rusks! It is actually very tasty!! Never thought it to be possible! Well, here goes:

500 grams melted butter
2 cups rice flour
2 cups potato flour/potato starch
10ml Himalayan salt
1 cup brown sugar (if you like sweet rusks, you can add a little more
        sugar … I think one cup is just enough)
½ cup psyllium husk
500 ml gluten free oats or normal oats if your body is OK with oats
2 teaspoons vanilla essence
10 teaspoons gluten free baking powder

½ to full cup sunflower seeds or pumpkin seeds (I prefer pumpkin)
½ to full cup desiccated coconut (based on your preference)
3 free range eggs
1 cup plain yogurt, full cream
500 ml buttermilk
1 cup dried cranberries or goji berries
         (I prefer goji berries – cranberries add to sweetness)
1 cup shredded cashew nuts (You can use other nuts of you prefer)

Method:

Mix all the ingredients. The mix should not be too wet not too dry, add yogurt if too dry or a bit flour if too wet. Rub you pans with some butter and press the dough into your pans. Bake until brown at 180°C, remove, cut to size, and put back into the oven to dry at 70°C until completely dry – approximately 5-6 hours. Now enjoy with a lovely cup of filter coffee!

Smoothies

My 'go to' smoothie consist of a teaspoon ground mixed nuts, a teaspoon rice protein powder, 3 table spoons plain yogurt, a handful blue berries, a few mint leaves and sage leaves, a spring onion, coconut cream to taste, a drop of honey and water – I enjoy it as a shake rather than a thick smoothie. I sometimes add a half banana or half an apple or any other fruit I have on hand.

Stew/Potjie

A stew is a great option. Add you favourite meats and veggies and use coconut milk instead of water. Ad you favourite organic spices and herbs.

Vanilla Chai Smoothie

Mix the following in your smoothie maker:
½ cup unsweetened almond or coconut milk
2 cups water

2-4 tablespoon ground seeds or nuts,
¼ teaspoon ground cinnamon
¼ tablespoon ground ginger
⅛ teaspoon ground cardamom
⅛ teaspoon ground cloves
Ice

Veggies

Use roasted veg mix. Boil until soft. Add coconut sugar with cinnamon when done. Coconut sugar and cinnamon adds amazing flavour to veggies.

For great gluten free recipe ideas, go to https://glutenfree onashoestring.com/

We've almost come to the end...before I close off practical guidance on where to start, I would like to share a small glimpse of my journey with you. Fasten your seatbelt!

Section 20

A Glimpse of my Journey

TURNING MY PAIN INTO PURPOSE

My greatest wealth is my health

A Glimpse of my journey...

It is March 2015. I am awaking after theatre. Just had a subtotal hysterectomy. I feel terrible. This is the most pain I have experienced in my whole life. But now I have to go through the motions. After years of recurring ovarian cysts my gynaecologist suggested a hysterectomy.

I get released from hospital and my Mom comes and stays with me as my husband is working in another town. For some reason I just can't get my strength back. Weeks pass. My Mom eventually goes home. I can't get out of bed in the morning and battle to get anything done during the day.

Luckily, I work from home and just finished a major contract, so if need be, I can rest when I have to. It gets worse. I feel like I am 100 years old, if not older. Going to the bathroom is an effort. Putting one foot in front of the other is agonising. Preparing food for myself is too much work. I am out of breath just to sit up straight in bed. It can't go on like this! On the 6th of March 2015 I visit my GP. He tells me it is stress and sends me on my merry way.

I felt helpless and decided to go back to my gynaecologist for a check-up. I am immediately admitted to hospital on the 18th of March 2015 and submitted to multiple blood tests, x-rays, ultrasound and scans. My gynaecologist introduces me to a physician who after all his tests confirms that I have Graves' Disease. This explained my elevated heart rate. For weeks it was between 110 – 140 beats per minute. One feels extremely fatigued when your heart rate goes that high. This is what doctors call hyper-thyriodism. Hypo-thyroidism on the other hand is when your thyroid is under active and your heart rate goes too slow. Both make you feel extremely tired.

He explained to me that my own immune system was attacking my thyroid. Consequently, I had an enlarged thyroid with nodules on it. Furthermore, he said that my options were (1) surgery, which he did not recommend as my vocal cords could be damaged, and (2) radio-active iodine which would basically shrink my thyroid and render it underactive.

In my ignorance, I went for the second option. Amazingly those were the only two options I was given. Little did I know there was a third option! Change your lifestyle!!

If any one of you out there are diagnosed with any autoimmune disease, I urge you to first seek help from an Integrative Health Practitioner.

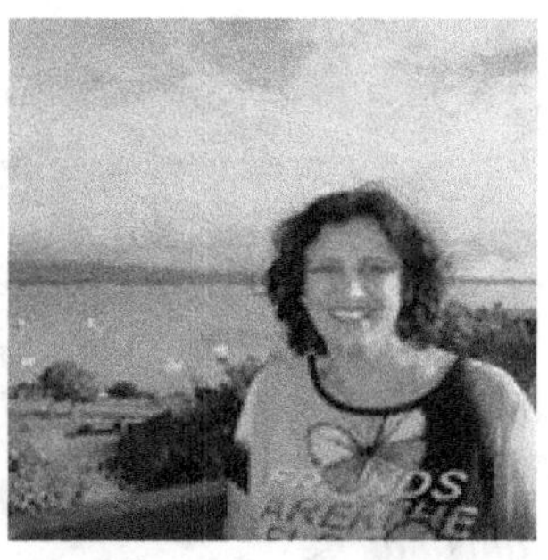

I met with the Nuclear Medicine Specialist. She explained to me that they would administer the radio-active iodine in the form of one single capsule specially prepared for me. She also said that radioiodine also has no known side effects (whatever!!!!!). I took this capsule on the 19th of March 2015, less than a week before my husband and I went overseas to visit my sister in New Zealand and for a short island holiday in Fiji. Up to the point that we landed in New Zeeland; I was still extremely fatigued. To my amazement I felt better whilst overseas. My body still took strain especially because we walked a lot. But I was able to enjoy my holiday.

The day after we came back, I woke up with my eyes swollen shut. My face looked like a soccer ball. For the next three months, I felt like I was climbing Mount Everest. Now my hyper thyroid turned hypo, and I was put on Eltroxin.

Medical Science turning a blind eye

I first called the physician who diagnosed me to explain my symptoms. His response was that swollen eyes are not likely to be as a result of my thyroid condition nor a side effect of the radioiodine. Besides the 10 minutes that I saw him in the hospital when he told me I had Graves; I never saw him again. He gave no advice as to any lifestyle or diet changes. His only advice was to go for radio-active iodine. I felt extremely frustrated and left alone in the dark.

The radio-active iodine was administered by a single capsule. I was told that it could work over the next 12 months to shrink my thyroid.

In my desperation I contacted the Nuclear Medicine specialist who administered the radioiodine, she told me she does not consult. I sent numerous e-mails begging for guidance and support. She just ignored it. Her assistant tried to answer but could not do so with confidence.

This is an extract of a mail I sent on the 7th of July 2015:

"Hi there, I would really appreciate if the Dr could give me some feedback. All I need to know is if the symptoms I have relate to my slow metabolism. Especially my eyes and general swelling, face, eyes, hands and feet. If so, I will wait for the eltroxin to work. If not, what should I do?

My GP just treats me for allergies...but also tells me my blood tests indicates no allergies.

I am at a loss

Thank you

Davida"

His response:

"Hi Mrs Van der Walt,

Sorry for not replying earlier.

Dr was unfortunately unavailable today. What I can tell you from my experience with previous patients is that most of your symptoms are similar to what our other patients have experienced. I will confirm with Dr first thing tomorrow morning and let you know.

     Your Greatest Wealth is your Health

Kind Regards,

Drs Assistant"

My response:

"Thank you so much. I am just so frustrated. Have been feeling like this for months and the Doctors think it is in my head.

I just need to know what to expect next and to do next

Thank you kindly

Davida"

His response:

Good Day Mrs Van der Walt,

I trust you are well.

Dr has prescribed Tertroxin for you for 5 days that you should take in conjunction with your Eltroxin. It is also a thyroid hormone that will help to make you feel a little better, faster. We will then still redo your blood tests in 4 weeks to check if the Eltroxin dosage is correct.

Kind Regards,

Drs Assistant"

Do note, she says nothing about my symptoms. It felt to me like I was ignored. From the pictures you can see how quickly I went from looking myself to looking like someone I did not know. In a matter of 2-3 months.

The added medication did nothing to improve my health. Not knowing what to do and thinking that my symptoms could perhaps be an allergy, I then went to another GP. I told him about my diagnoses and the radio-iodine treatment. He did blood test after blood test, but nothing! He gave me weekly antihistamine injections. It actually made me worse. After a few weeks he told me he can't help me as he can't find anything wrong with me. It must be in my head. His receptionist told me that when she drinks too much wine over a weekend her face also swells. I was so angry. At the time I was too sick to even consider a glass of wine. Needless to say, I never went back to him. This is what I looked like in June. I could not even recognise myself. By now I was so frustrated I could cry.

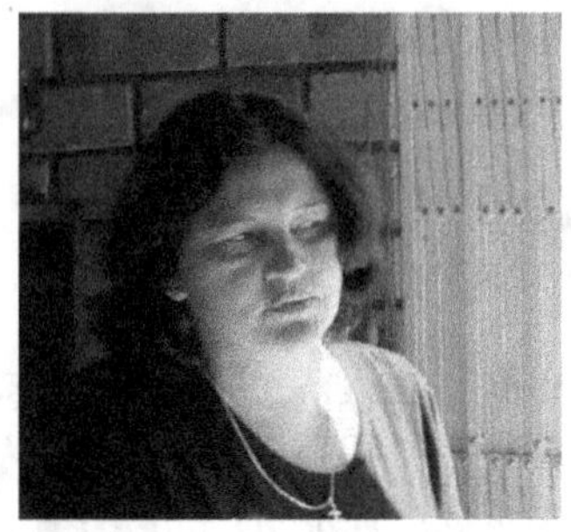

I felt horrible. I always felt tired and exhausted, I looked horrible, and I was extremely sensitive to everything. So much so that I could not figure out what. I at one stage thought I was allergic to fabric. Perhaps my pillow is the problem? I bought hypo-allergic pillowcases and bed covers. But nothing seemed to help.

In my desperation, I went to an Ophthalmologist on the 29th of May. He told me I have dry eyes. No luck there.

On the 28th of July 2015, I went to see another eye specialist, hoping they would know something about Graves. This doctor told me about a friend of hers that is going through the same thing, but she could not provide me with any answers.

By now I felt lost...at this stage I would rather die than carry on like this. Waking up feeling horrible, no energy, swollen beyond recognition. Reacting to everything and battling to find out just exactly what I am reacting to.

I did some more research on Graves and realised it may help to see an endocrinologist. I started doing web searches looking for endocrinologists who specialise in thyroid conditions. I found a site which had references. I found a doctor that came highly recommended. My first appointment was 17 August 2016. This doctor spent almost an hour with me, listening to what symptoms I experienced and interacting with me. I was so relieved! He suggested a magnitude of blood tests which I gladly did. (None of which the GP did).

     Your Greatest Wealth is your Health

He found that my TSH Receptor Antibodies were very high. It was 248 at the time. Normal ranges below 1.8. This explained my severe chemical sensitivities and lack of ability to lose weight. He helped me get my Eltroxin at the correct levels to avoid being either hyper or hypo. It took months to stabilise. He also started me on DHEA and significant doses of Vitamin D3.

In November 2015, I started having severe swelling of my feet. Actually, my whole body was inflamed, swollen and sore...but my feet took the brunt of it. I love exercise, what got to me was that I could never exercise. The moment I tried to do a brisk walk or run; my feet would swell so severely that I could not walk. I remember going shopping, before we even enter the store I could barely walk. I would always push the trolley as it would support me.

In December 2015, I did some more of my own research. (I actually never stopped, to this day!). I came across Low Dose Naltrexone (LDN). I asked my Endocrinologist if he would prescribe me LDN which he did. It had a remarkable effect on my health. My Endocrinologist suggested I go off gluten and sugar. Both these steps also made a big difference.

This is a note I sent my Dr after starting to take LDN: *"Within 2 days after taking LDN I felt great. The swelling in my face and feet went right down for one whole day .... after that it started fluctuating again. I also have severe fluctuations in my energy levels and my pulse is going up. It used to be 60 on average...in the last week it went up to 90 and have now seem to have settled on 70. I still feel confident that I should just carry on and see what happens...I guess any changes in my hormone levels, even good changes will cause symptoms."*

His response: *"Yes worthwhile to continue. If symptoms still persist after 12 weeks check your thyroid levels as you may need a dosage adjustment."*

What I really appreciated was his willingness to interact with me via e-mail. Whenever I had fluctuations in symptoms, I would e-mail him and ask for his advice. He always responded.

My research also guided me to take Omega 3 fish oils, as well as selenium and probiotics. I started using these religiously (self-prescribed).

My eye swelling remained a major issue. I also developed sores around my eyes (and on my neck and my head). I was so embarrassed, I started wearing dark shades just to hide my eyes. Can you see the bulge towards the right of my eye, that was swelling? It looked like a bag full of water.

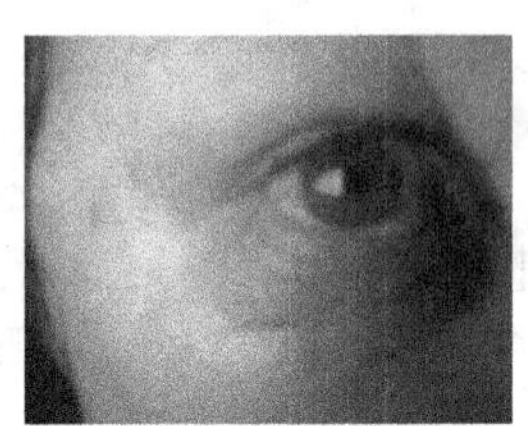

In November 2015, my Endocrinologist referred me to a Professor who specialises in Thyroid Eye Disease (TED). After his examination, he confirmed that I did not have Thyroid Eye Disease and that there was no permanent damage to my eyes. He could, however, not explain the severe swelling and soreness. Over and above the fact that my eyes were severely swollen, they were also extremely dry and always very sore. And extremely light sensitive. It did not take much for me to strain my eyes. I do a lot of computer work and at times had to stop working to give my eyes a break.

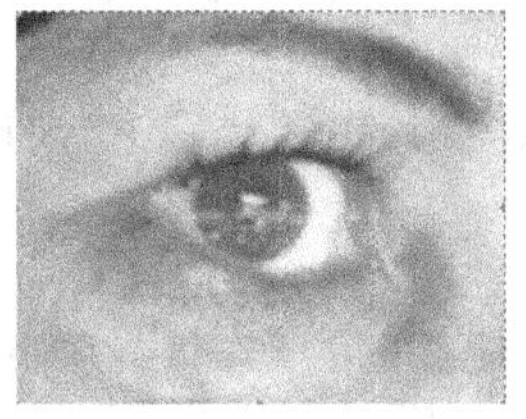

In my continuous search for answers, I 'hesitantly' saw a Dr in Ethnomedicine.[1][2] This was February 2016. Below a photo of what my blood looked like at the time. Blood cells should look like marbles. Round. Not like this!

This Doctor said there were mycoplasma in my blood.[3]

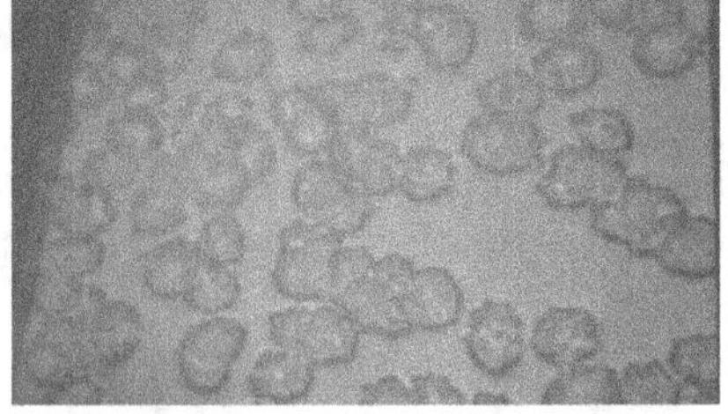

He prescribed olive leaf extract and folic acid. After taking his prescribed medicine, I initially felt worse. I actually wrote him an e-mail where I explained that it felt to me as if something was boiling me from the inside.

What actually happened was that I detoxed too fast. My body was extremely toxic, in which case the release of toxins had to be managed. I also later did a detox which made me completely ill. If you are finding yourself in the same position, remember to take it slow. Exercise and mild detox are the best remedy, but it does take time. Be patient and be kind to yourself.

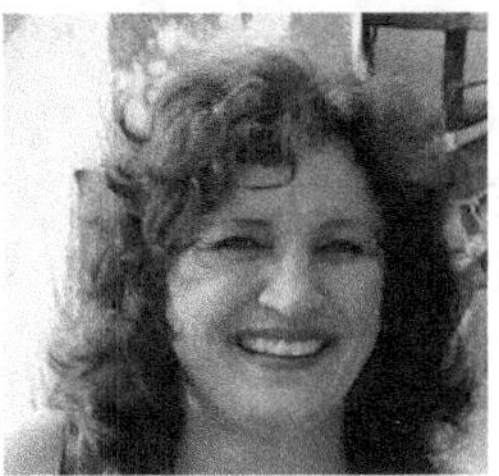

A natural product that I felt helped a lot was Dandelion Root Extract Tea. Whenever I have severe chemical sensitivities, I would drink a pot of tea and it relieved my symptoms almost immediately.

In the next few months my blood results improved, but I still felt swollen, sore and fatigued. And I gained weight!

I furthered my research and learned about the devastating effect of food choices and environmental toxins on my body. I started implementing all the measures explained in this book. One at a time. It took me many years of research to put it all together. I started swimming, one lap at first, and slowly I increased my exercise. Today I hike an average of 1 hour a day on a mountain top.

I kept up seeing my Endocrinologist throughout the year 2016. He asked me to keep up the lifestyle changes as these started to render great results. Removing gluten from my diet made a huge difference. Once I was able to exercise, this made an even bigger difference.

In May 2016 it felt like I had a huge Adams Apple, which I never had before. I caught a big fright and was sent to a surgeon. After a scan, it was established that all was good. The doctor said it could be that the radioiodine that is literally shrinking my thyroid, is now exposing more bone in my throat.

That was my last big scare...I am continuing my research...I don't think I will ever stop. There is always something more we can learn.

In 2017 I started seeing a Functional Medicine Practitioner who helped me identify natural supplements that could help over that last hurdle. This was done based on extensive blood tests that are not standard for your mainstream medical practitioners.

If you have an autoimmune disease, I urge you to see a Functional Medical Practitioner.

Great Resources on my Journey

For interest sake, Dr Eric Osansky was the first site I stumbled on which had a major impact on my health.

He has multiple free webinars and resources. He talks to the link between thyroid and cholesterol. http://www.naturalendocrine solutions.com/free-webinars/

Through his blogs, he introduced me to Magdalena Wszelaki. She's a certified nutrition coach, and after having the antibodies for both Graves' Disease and Hashimoto's, she was able to restore her health, and over the years she has been helping people with endocrine conditions balance their hormones through the use of whole, healthy foods.

From there I started following Dr Tom O'Bryan, Dr Mark Hyman, Dr Osborne, Naomi Whittel, Dr Jay Davidson, Eric Zielinski, Jonathan Otto, Wendy Myers, Dr Axe, Dr Z, James Maskell, Green Smoothie Girl, Dr Alan Christianson, Nicole Hunn, Evan Brand, Mike Adams, Dr Michael Murray, Sayer Ji at GreenMedInfo, and many more quoted in this programme. Let me just say, these are trusted sources!

The key messages by all these wonderful people are:

1. Keep your gut clean (cut gluten and sugar, and eat whole foods)
2. Support your liver
3. Balance your sugar
4. Remove as many environmental toxins as you can
5. Actively manage your stress
6. And keep moving!

What are the signs I missed over the years?

Interestingly enough, I have always thought I followed a "healthy" lifestyle. I believed in eating healthy foods and exercise. I have also throughout my life developed and implemented stress management strategies.

But for about 5-10 years before I was diagnosed, I did not feel well. I would wake up in the morning with very sore feet. It was so swollen I could barely walk. I always thought that my feet first needed to warm up and then I could go full steam. The second major symptom was fatigue. My feet always felt warm, like a burning sensation.

Then there were swollen glands, an inflamed jaw, headaches, severe constipation, endometriosis, burning feet, acid reflux, hives, allergies, chemical sensitivities, strained eyes and eye sight fluctuations, muscle aches and pains, a very oily skin (today it is normal), lack of concentration, memory loss, mood swings, fever, blood sugar drops, hair loss, ear infection and brain fog.

I had endless ovarian cysts, one after the other. I would get these fever spells, where my body felt like it wanted to burn out. These were toxins fighting to get out of my body!

It was a host of general, vague symptoms. I remember talking to my husband about having kids. I told him that I just could not see myself having kids the way I felt. The GP told me I am stressed and after seeing a specialist, I was told I have fibromyalgia. I refused to believe it. I am not a depressed person, nor do I have fibromyalgia. Now, years later, I realise my healthy lifestyle was not so healthy.

Ironically, I always ate rye bread, thinking it is healthier that white or brown bread. Little did I know what havoc the gluten wreaked in my body.

What I thought was a healthy lifestyle, wasn't the case. I can't blame myself; I did not know of any better. Few people out there know what I know. I sincerely hope that going through this programme will open your eyes.

Whilst I was in recovery, in my ignorance, with the little I knew at that stage(in January 2016) I sent my Endocrinologist this mail – I think you will appreciate this:

For your interest, I have made you a list of the challenges I experience from day to day and how I cope with them (feel free to share them with patients going through the same as I am)

Exercise with caution

I can for instance not exercise. If I do, my feet swell severely. I do gentle swimming which makes me feel energised.

Bruising

I bruise easily. When I get mosquito bites, I need to be very careful not take all my skin off when I scratch. I need to be very aware of scratching as gently as possible.

Dry eyes

My eyes are extremely dry. It has improved quite a bit over the last year, but still remains a challenge. I have to be very careful with fans and air conditioners. As a rule, I always have artificial tear drops close to me and use to frequently throughout the day. Gel drops work really well.

Swelling all over

The worst effect is on my eyes and my feet. When I was at my worst, before making diet changes, I looked like a different person. My hands also swell, especially my fingers. When I eat really well (in other words no sugar or gluten), it improves. And I need to drink a lot of water. During the colder months, it poses a real challenge, as drinking water is far easier to do in the summer.

Food impacts my health

I need to be super careful what I eat. Omitting sugar and gluten from your diet is the best remedy. When I eat processed food that contains sugar and or gluten, I become very fatigued and the swelling kicks in almost immediately and takes anything from 1-3 days to settle. I say settle, cause it never really goes away, it is just the extent that differs. I do eat gluten free bread and sugar free chocolates. It is amazing how creative one can get if you need to. I enjoy freshly made veggie juices (without cruciferous veggies as they impact the thyroid), and a daily plain yogurt smoothie with dark berries.

Alcoholic and sugary drinks cause havoc

The same goes for drinking alcohol. I personally love a glass of wine. For some time, I was not able to drink anything but water and herbal tea. Now I can enjoy a glass of dry wine once a week. I find that dry wine has the least effect. In moderation that is! I have now developed a habit to drink rooibos tea first thing in the morning. I also enjoy freshly made ginger tea with a little bit of honey. I drink 1-2 cups of decaf coffee a day and limit my caffeine intake.

Long distance travelling is a nightmare

If I sit for long periods, I become extremely stiff and start swelling. We recently had a road trip that took 9 hours.... within the first hour I felt the swelling increasing. By the time we got to our destination, my feet were swollen badly. It is especially bad when I travel higher than sea level. By switching on the air conditioner and setting the cold air to direct to my feet does help somewhat.

Pushing myself is a no no

Pacing myself is a skill I had to learn over the last year. I have always been able to push myself to the limits and beyond. Should I do that now, I would just collapse and mean nothing to no one. I can push myself quite hard for a day or two, and then need to slow down considerably the next day or two by perhaps sleeping late or going to bed early and reducing the amount of work I do in a day. By pacing myself, I am able to deliver at a constant rate.

     Your Greatest Wealth is your Health

Feeling lethargic

The first thought that comes to my mind when I wake up is the pain in my feet and legs, and an intoxicated feeling in my head. It literally feels like a hangover. More often than not I wake in the morning feeling like I want to turn on my side, pull the covers over my head and sleep some more. By doing so I run the risk of falling onto depression. It is not an option!! I simply get up, get ready and start working at whatever pace my body allows. This approach has kept me motivated and able to go on. I found that moving my body, walking, swimming or any movement, increases my blood flow and actually makes me feel better. Not moving at all keeps me in that low energy state where I do not feel like doing anything. It is critical to get moving, feeling better and getting on with it!

The body does not always want to work with me

I have to listen to my body. Some days are just much worse than others. This goes with pacing myself. This morning I woke up feeling drained. I actually did sleep an extra 2 hours and then got up, got myself moving and I actually felt better. When my body retaliates severely, I listen, I pace myself, but never stop moving! Do not push your body over its limits, it does far more harm than good.

Low blood sugar causes terrible symptoms

A fairly easy strategy, but equally critical, is keeping my blood sugar stable. The moment my blood sugar is unstable, I feel fatigued and just generally ill. When I get up in the morning, after taking my eltroxin, I eat immediately after an hour has transpired. If I skip breakfast or eat breakfast later in the morning, I feel terrible. I eat small amounts at least every two hours. It keeps my blood sugar and energy levels stable.

Tight shoes or clothes are a no-no

I love my jeans but can't wear them. Any tight-fitting clothes increases the swelling. The same goes for shoes. I can't wear any shoes such as running shoes, boots or any shoe that fits tightly around my feet.

Not enough sleep is not an option

If I do not get enough sleep, I wake up more swollen than usual, pain in my eyes, and a general feeling of sickness. A sound 8-hour sleep routine makes a big difference.

Weight gain...well yes

I have gained 10kg over the last year and have no way to lose it. My Doctor has advised me that until my TSH Receptor Antibodies are close to zero, my weight will remain a challenge.

Environmental toxins are killers

I am super sensitive to any toxins. Perfume, toilet spray, pool chemicals, hair colour, you name it. I now use bio-friendly household products, hair colour without ammonia, and furthermore I avoid any strong perfumes or toxins of any nature. If I expose myself to it, I feel horrible!! When my husband applies deodorant, he leaves our bedroom and sprays it on in a different room in the house, and then closes that door until the fumes subsided.

Standing or sitting still is a challenge

When I sit for extended periods, which I need to do often as most of my work is computer-based, I get very stiff and swollen. The same for standing still in one place. It is not a nice experience. As long as I move around often and allow for some blood circulation, I feel much better. I think that the excess TSH receptor antibodies act as a severe toxin in my body.

Today I have moved so far beyond the state I described above...I eat cruciferous veggies on a daily basis, I exercise at least an hour for 5 days a week, I avoid gluten like the plague, I drink at least 2 litres water a day, I pace myself, and when I have to work extra hard, I build in recovery time, I sleep well and create an environment where I can sleep well, I get fresh air and sun spending time in nature, I judge less and love more, I pray a lot, I live 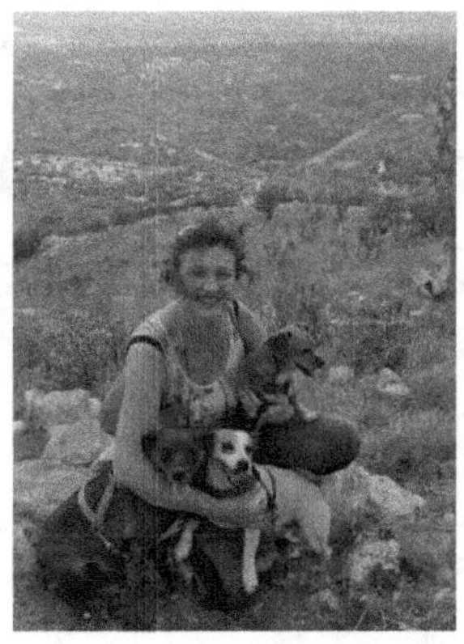 gratefully, I live my passion, I regularly do intermittent fasting, and yes I love to eat, so I make an effort to find awesome gluten free recipes! Anything from moist chocolate cake to delicious black bean brownies. I do not deprive myself! And best of all, I feel great, look good, and have the energy to do what I want...what a blessing! I mostly eat organic and free range, not always possible, but I try. And I do not feel guilty when I do not manage to do so. I know which foods I can cheat with and which I should avoid at all cost. So, if I wish to cheat some, I do it wisely. I know my body, and I listen to my body. By making these changes, all my symptoms and illnesses mysteriously vanished! ☺

One of the biggest lessons I have learned is that one needs to still live! What can you do to avoid feeling deprived? You need to figure this out for yourself.... Here you can see my transformation – I bet you can't believe it is the same person. So here I am, turning my pain into my purpose:

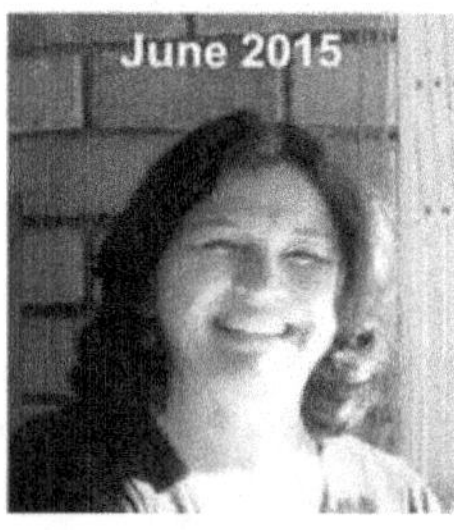

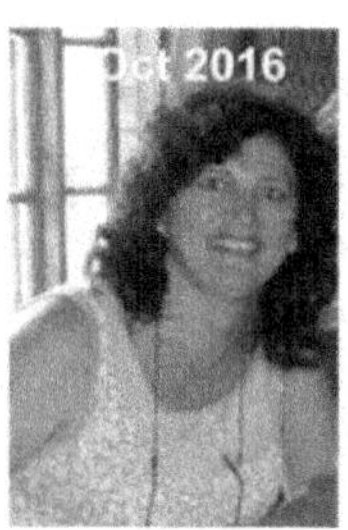

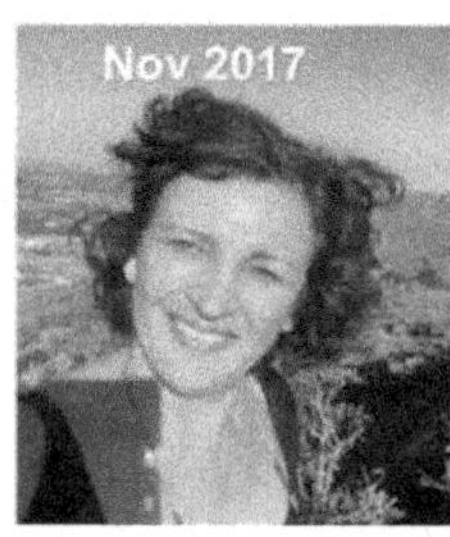

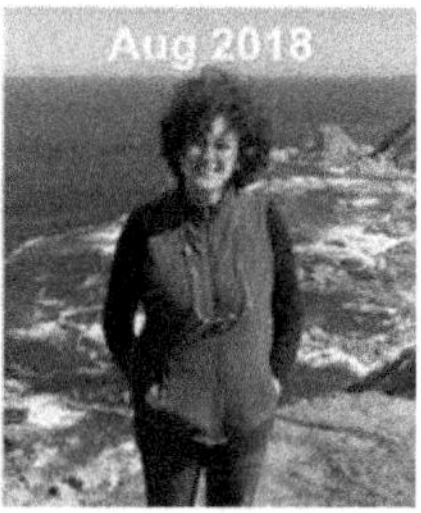

I thought to give you a glimpse of what I went through. I am sure many of you will be able to relate. Now it is your turn to take the bull by the horns and make the changes that will change your life!!

REMEMBER, YOUR GREATEST WEALTH IS YOUR HEALTH!

Now it is your turn!

Sources of References in Section 20

1. http://www.thyroid-info.com/articles/brownstein.htm
2. http://www.drgregemerson.com/fact-file/mycoplasma
3. http://www.rense.com/general62/molecularterrorism.htm

Section 21
In summary – What now?

NOW YOU TAKE CHARGE
OF YOUR HEALTH

When all is said and done...time for action

Rebecca Coomes, with her 5 Pillars to Health summarises the core of this programme beautifully:[1]

1. **Raise your Awareness** – reconnect with your body...listen to the signals (moods, allergies etc)

2. **Nourish your body through good Nutrition** – we are what we eat. Be aware of what you are eating.

3. **Get moving** – especially when we don't feel well. Movement in gentle way, not necessarily a marathon. Step away from the PC and move.

4. **Keep your Mindset in check** – be aware not to be negative. Think positively.

5. **Follow a Lifestyle conducive to health.**

I would like to add two bullets:

6. **Detox your external environment** – get rid of all those toxic substances in your life that are putting strain on your body

7. **Detox from toxic relationships**

Following these few simple steps can revolutionise your life.

The whole aim is to follow a lifestyle that will slowly but surely detox your body from excess toxin build-up, but also ensure that your body in future is not overloaded with toxins. It is an approach to proactive detox as a lifestyle rather than radical detox.

The following organs can be supported to detox as described below:

Skin	Exercise (sweating), dry brushing, using natural products on your skin, following a healthy, clean, organic, whole food diet
Kidneys	Drinking sufficient clean water, eating organic fruit in moderation, eating berries (cranberries, black cherries, blue berries), making wise choices with regards to alcohol, caffeine and chocolate, consuming dandelion tea, eating beets and spinach, drinking water with freshly squeezed lemon juice first thing in the morning
Liver	Remove toxic and inflammatory foods from your diet, eating raw veggies, natural supplements such as milk thistle, dandelion and turmeric
Colon	Avoiding foods you have intolerances for, eating foods loaded with pre-and probiotics, eating high fiber foods/veggies that keeps you regular, eating fermented foods, eating fresh organic fruits, especially berries or apples which contain pectin fiber, consuming bone broth, consuming healthy fats like coconut or avocados. Colon cleanses or coffee enemas can also be of use.
Lungs	Clean air (getting out in nature), deep breathing, eating fresh herbs like ginger, oregano and peppermint (great for making teas), improving the air quality in your home, quit smoking (if you are a smoker), limit or remove dairy from your diet, drink green tea, drink carrot juice, take a hot bath or shower, make use of eucalyptus oil in a diffuser, exercise.
Lymphatic system	Dry brushing, regular exercise, rebounding, massage, eating a variety of fruits and raw veggies (if you can tolerate), yoga, drink lots of clean water, eating lots of fresh herbs such as garlic, ginger and turmeric, deep breathing, using natural deodorant, doing hydrotherapy (alternating warm and cold water in your morning shower), sauna of steam bath, avoid wearing tight clothes.

Please stop and read the above table again!! This information can transform your life!!!

Reality is you need a detox, and a quick 7-day detox won't cut it. You need to make lifestyle changes that will detox your body but also keep your body clean. These are summarised in this table. Please go back and read it again!

I hope this table provides you with a nice concise summary of habits that could transform your health!

Now where do we start? The easiest way is to start with your diet.

Remember, everything you eat either causes inflammation or reduces inflammation!

This means you need to start thinking about what you eat. Do not just grab the first thing you can put your hands on. Think about the effect of food on your body!

One small change can have a massive impact. Remember to combine proteins with healthy fats and fiber. Do not try and do it all at the same time. Under no circumstances can you allow yourself to be overwhelmed. Toxins are a reality but making one small change can have a massive impact on your health and that of your family.

It was mentioned before that the easiest, most effective way to confirm if you have any allergies or food intolerances, is to eliminate these from your diet and see what happens. I would like to recommend that you first remove the following from your diet as part of the process of elimination:

1. All Gluten / Grains (incl corn)
2. Alcohol [2] (It wreaks havoc on your brain, heart, liver, pancreas and immune system – do read the article in the link provided)
3. Dairy

4. Processed sugar

Take these one at a time. Remove them for three weeks and if you wish to reintroduce to see what happens, introduce one at a time and wait at least 3 days to see if you have any negative symptoms. DO NOT INTRODUCE MORE THAN ONE AT A TIME. Remember, this is a journey!

Rather take your time and tackle one at a time. That way you will not be overwhelmed with the changes, and you will know for sure what affects you.

Together with your diet, intermittent fasting can help you accelerate your healing. Try the 16/8 model three days a week…not consecutive days, rather every second day. What works well for most people is to start on a Sunday evening, let's say having a last meal at 17h00, then eating at 9h00 again on the Monday…then eating normally until Tuesday evening. Again, have your last meal let's say at 18h00 and eat at 10h00 the next morning. And the same again from Thursday evening to Friday morning. Taking the weekend off is perfectly fine. This you have to try. ***Do not fast every day!!*** Your body also needs a break…You could though, on a permanent basis, fast three days a week on the 16/8 principle.

Once you have settled on the above, you can start eliminating the following (one at a time):

1. Eggs
2. Legumes
2. Night shade vegetables
3. Soy
4. Nuts
5. Shell fish

By default, you need to reduce your sugar intake, and avoid all deep-fried foods, processed foods or snacks, preservatives, colourants and food additives. You can try doing a food intolerance test using the elimination diet, but I can promise you that your body will respond negatively to these foreign invaders. They are not good for you!

Make a decision today to go for whole foods.

By eating whole foods, you do not have to think about what you can or can't eat. Now isn't that making it easy! It automatically cuts out the bad stuff and introduces the good stuff. But remember to eat a nice variety of foods of different colours.

Dr Terry Wahls recovered from Multiple Sclerosis after being in a wheelchair for 4 years.[3] She did this with major diet and lifestyle changes. She recommends 8-9 cups of veggies a day! She now treats people with autoimmune diseases.

She says the phytonutrients contained in veggies have a major impact on health improvement.

When she works with patients, she requires that they follow her programme 100% for 100 days. That includes amongst other, removing harmful foods such as sugar, grains, legumes and night shade veggies, and adding 9 cups veggies a day to the diet. I love that she does this. Her results are remarkable. Are you getting this?! Eat more veggies! You will feel and see the difference!

This is a very important rule of thumb: Variety and Colour!

Mike Geary reports that the foods that are worst for your brain are fructose trans fats, mercury and wheat-based foods.

He says many so-called health products are loaded with concentrated fructose. Natural whole fruits do contain fructose, but generally contain MUCH smaller quantities of fructose than you would consume in a sweetened juice drink, soft drink or sweetened junk foods. Also, the phytonutrients, antioxidants, and fiber that's contained in most whole fruits counteracts any negative effects of fructose. I personally try to keep fruit intake to no more than 1-2 pieces a day due to the sugar and fructose content of larger amounts of fruit. Low GI fruits include berries and granny smith apples.

The easiest way to approach this section is by eating a great variety of vegetables of different colours! The key is moderation and variety!!

Too much of anything is not good for you!! Except for veggies, as long as you eat a variety!! The last thing you want to do is only eat one or two apparently good foods, and it ends up doing you harm because you eat too much of it.

To simplify your choices, go to the supermarket, and buy a mix of veggies of different colours, and eat those. If at first, these are not organic, it is still better than not eating veggies! As you grow into your new habits, you can consider growing your own veggies in your garden or buying organic from your farmers market. Just start somewhere.

Cruciferous veggies are amazing!! They will help you detox, and you will feel the difference. Just start eating them. And remember, add colour to your diet! And remember to add extra water intake to your daily routine.

And I want to remind you, a single change can change your world and your health.[4]

The best bit of advice I can give you is to not buy the culprits. Stock your fridge with the good stuff.

And experiment with great recipes that are gluten free, or perhaps sugar or dairy free. There is so much available on the internet. In Section 18, I provide you with some ideas. Check out the snack ideas!!

We all need a crutch. That crutch is a delicious snack recipe that is high in protein and healthy fats but tastes just as nice as your favourite sweet or snack. Check out Section 18 for ideas.

Always remember that fruit juices contain high levels of fructose and should be avoided unless significantly diluted.

Trans fats, as we discussed before, are found in all hydrogenated oils, processed foods and deep-fried foods.

Soy sauce can be a bugger if you are intolerant. It also contains gluten. I cut it from my diet for months. Then one Sunday we decided to go for Chinese, loaded with soy sauce, the next morning I could not get out of bed. Organic tamari is a great substitute. **Be careful of these seemingly innocent offenders.**

Mercury is found in tuna. If you suspect mercury toxicity, rather eat salmon and avoid tuna for a while. And avoid eating any foods from tins.

Throw out the margarine, and rather eat butter in moderation.

Remember to make your food interesting. Add fresh garlic, ginger, oregano or any other fresh herbs and spices.

Wheat based foods have been dealt with at length. Besides the fact that it damages your gut lining, wheat contains compounds termed "exorphins" that have an effect in your brain similar to opiate drugs. It is addictive. This explains why people have such a hard time giving up their breads, cereals, pasta, and muffins. If you enjoy bread, make sure to check out Nature's Choice Crusty Four Flour Bread Pre-Mix or Glutagon's Soft White Bread Pre-Mix. Both these breads are amazing.

The moral of the story is, cut these "bad" foods from your diet and see what happens!

The message is that if you really want to be well (healthy in the true sense of the word), compromising won't get you there.

Remember to eat a high protein breakfast, with healthy fats and fiber. Easy options are an egg with an avo or an omelette with veggies, made with coconut milk. My personal favourite is a smoothie with coconut milk, plain yogurt, water, blue berries, ground seeds and nuts, natural protein powder, and some green leafy veggies.

Remember the blue berries.

Remember your blue berries. Buy these frozen, in bulk, and add to your smoothies, eat as a snack, or add it to your gluten free baking.

It must be said at this time that making lifestyle changes is not always easy. It takes a lot of commitment and dedication.

You will be faced with endless social pressure to go back to your old ways. The first weekend you spend with friends they will say: "Come on, have a glass of wine with me…". Stand your ground, take some home-made iced tea, or water with some ground ginger and a bit of honey, or water flavoured with fresh mint and sliced lemon, or some coconut water. Reducing alcohol intake to reduce inflammation in your body is a key step. You will be able to enjoy a drink again, but while your body is chronically inflamed, you are just pouring oil on the fire.

You may also be your own worst enemy! Food addiction is just as bad as drug addiction. Food releases the same hormones in your brain as addictive drugs do. The most practical way to address these food urges, is to ensure you clean out your cupboards and remove all temptation. Get rid of products loaded with gluten, preservatives, additives and so forth. Make sure your house is stocked with healthy alternatives. This includes healthy snacks.

Do remember to introduce prebiotic and probiotic loaded foods and anti-inflammatory foods into your diet.

Make sure you don't feel deprived! Experiment with great foods and snacks!

This is a major success factor. Play around with the recipes provided and find what works for you.

To make a success of your diet changes, preparation is a MUST!

If you prepare your meals on a weekly basis and freeze them, it becomes much easier to just grab something from the freezer and warm it up. My go to meal is a bean meal. Over weekends I soak my beans overnight and cook them soft the next day. I fry some onion, chicken mince, peppers, or whatever veggies I have in the fridge. Add some fresh garlic and ginger, and there you go! I freeze these in suitable portions in glass containers. Other great freezing options are bobotie, potjie and soup. I use coconut milk in all my meals, instead of water.

Similarly, I buy bulk coconut flakes and prepack them in small portions. I also make my black bean brownies, date balls and home-made chocolates. If I battle to eat healthy fats with my meals, I just eat a chocolate with my meal. I avoid buying chocolates, which forces me to eat my own home-made chocolates. And trust me, they taste great!

Another key dietary change would be to reduce your coffee intake. It is best to drink quality filter coffee. Get a small plunger which limits you to a single cup. The rest of the day enjoy your tea with a cinnamon stick and a star aniseed. Or add some honey. You will love the taste! Make a pot at a time and enjoy.

If you are one of those people who battle to drink water, flavour your water with cucumber, ginger, lemon or mint. Or a mix thereof. Or even blue berries.

Over and above your dietary changes, you need to get moving! Whatever movement your body can withstand. Just start somewhere, even if it means walking to the gate of your house and back. Listen to your body, start small and slowly increase your movement as the inflammation in your body subsides.

If you suspect any underlying infections, engage a functional medical practitioner or your homeopath.[5][6]

Start getting rid of your environmental toxins. Do not be overwhelmed, start with one at a time. I would recommend you start with changing your washing detergent to bicarbonate of soda (baking soda), and your toothpaste to a fluoride free toothpaste. Thereafter you can tackle them one at a time.

Keep your thoughts in check. Consciously start changing your thinking to be positive and uplifting.

Limit your exposure to EMF.

And lastly, introduce those life changing lifestyle changes such as deep breathing, being out in nature, grounding, taking frequent breaks, engaging in hobbies of your choice, spending quality time with family and friends and so forth.

Resist all the social pressures, stand your ground, and start making changes that will enhance your quality of life! Soon everyone will want to know what your secret is, and they will follow your lead.

How can one achieve this goal of living a healthy lifestyle for life? It is so important that you know why you are doing this?

Do you want to walk again? Do you want to be pain free? Do you want to enjoy a day of fun with the family without having to pull out because you are not feeling well? Do you want to lose weight? Do you want more energy? Do you want clarity of thought? Do you want to run 10 miles with a smile on your face and no pain?

I do not know what your motivation is. Mine was to live a normal life, to feel good and have the energy to do what I want. And to be pain free! (Which I can proudly say I am!)

I refuse to go back to where I was. I remember waking up not being able to walk. My feet being so swollen, that it took me at least 30 minutes before I could walk normally. I could not go shopping with my husband, because my feet were too swollen. If I did manage to get to the store, I would hang on to the shopping trolley to support me to walk through the store. I would look in the mirror and my eyes and face would be so swollen. I was embarrassed to meet people. I would wake up, my first thought being an acute awareness of the pain my body was in. And, when I went to sleep, that same acute awareness haunted my mind. I would work for an hour and would not be able to keep my eyes open. Fatigue would overshadow my whole being. Now that I know what is possible, I will only improve my health even further.

I am not prepared to compromise by eating cake at a birthday party unless it is gluten free. I refuse to go back to being in pain and battling to see through my eyes because of the pain in my eye sockets. I refuse! I want to be healthy and I want to be happy. I want to enjoy life!

Now if I am invited to a tea party, I take a platter of gluten free cake with. And everyone respects it. And quite frankly, if they don't, that is not my problem. ☺

In summary I would like to leave you with this graphic:

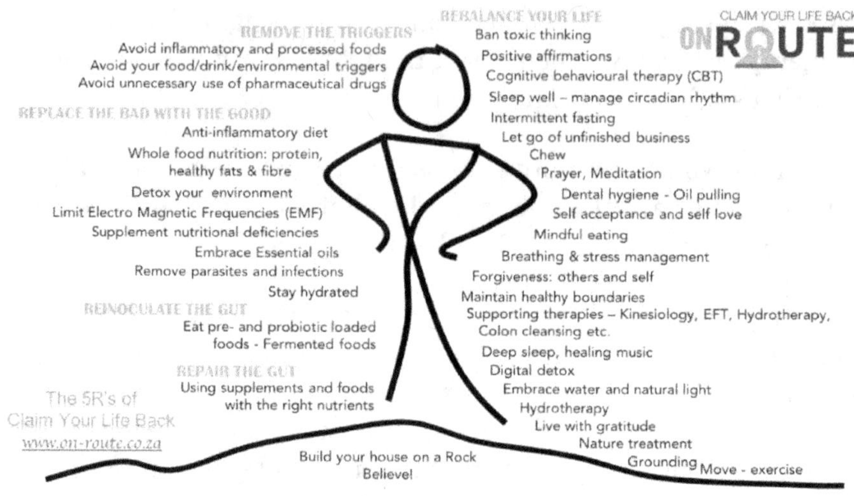

Apply the 5Rs in your life. Start somewhere, and slowly fill the gaps.

But if you wish to make a success of your journey, you need to know why you are entering into this programme and keep that goal in front of you. Do not lose sight of your goal and ultimately your motivation!

God designed our bodies to cope with toxins. Our bodies are masterfully designed to have multiple detox pathways to help us cope with our daily toxicity load. What am I saying? I do not want you to be in despair that you won't be able to conquer this "thing"! If you do your part to reduce your toxic load, your body's natural defences will kick in.

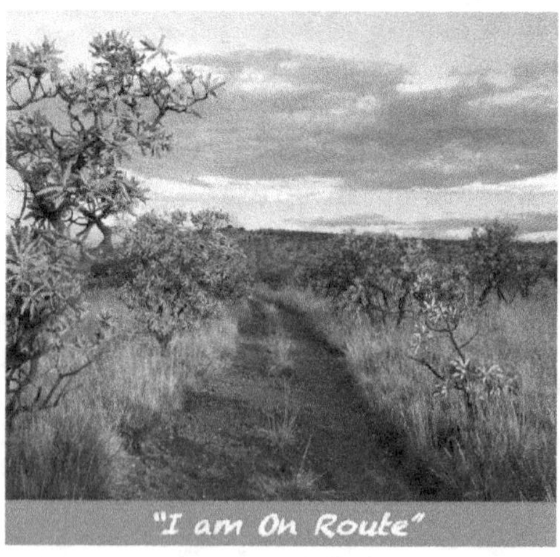

I mentioned in Section 1 that engaging in this programme is a journey. Each of us need to figure out what our triggers are...what our trigger foods are, what our trigger environmental toxins are, and what our emotional triggers are? You will each define your own journey. My hope and sincere wish for you is that this programme will guide you on that path.

You can do this! One step at a time, one day at a time!

Sources of References in Section 21

1. https://healthygutexperts.com/day-5/rebecca-coomes/
2. https://www.niaaa.nih.gov/publications/brochures-and-fact-sheets/hangovers
3. http://integrativewomenshealthinstitute.com/pelvic-pain-autoimmune-disease-dr-terry-wahls/
4. http://www.truthaboutabs.com/brain-harming-foods.html
5. https://dhesmed.com/dr-dhesan-g-moodley/
6. http://www.imcmed.co.za/mr-david-arthur/

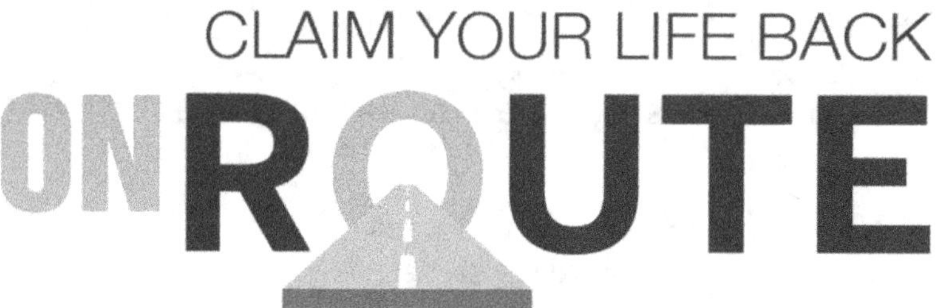

For more information, feel free to visit my website:

www.on-route.co.za

DISCLAIMER - The information provided in the Claim Your Life Back Programme and the book No More Illness, is for general information purposes and educational purposes only, aimed at improving lifestyle choices. All information is provided in good faith, however we make no representation or warranty of any kind, express or implied, regarding accuracy, adequacy, validity, availability or completeness of any information.

Under no circumstance shall we have any liability to you. The Programme does not contain any medical advice. Accordingly, before taking any actions based upon such information, we encourage you to consult with the appropriate medical professionals. The use or reliance of any information contained in the Programme is solely at your own risk.

9 781710 182958